Power, Politics, and Public Policy: A Matter of Caring

Edited by
Anne Boykin

National League for Nursing Press • New York
Pub. No. 14-2684

Copyright © 1995
National League for Nursing Press
350 Hudson Street, New York, NY 10014

ISBN: 0-88737-644-4

This book was set in Goudy by Publications Development Company. The edi-
tor was Maryan Malone. Northeastern Press was the printer and binder. The
cover was designed by Lauren Stevens.

Printed in the United States of America.

This book is dedicated
to the members of the International Association for Human Caring
and to all nurses whose commitment to caring
grounds their practice of nursing
and thereby directs choices;

and

to those persons who are willing to take the risks
and face the challenges necessary to address a societal mandate
for humanism.

A. B.

Contents

Preface   vii
    Anne Boykin
Peer Reviewers   ix
Contributors   xi
Introduction   xiii
    Tim Porter-O'Grady, EdD, PhD, FAAN
Caring Connections   xix
    Malcolm R. MacDonald

Part I   Power, Politics, and Public Policy: The Theory Lens   1

1.   The Dominant Paradigm of the Modern World   3
    Sister M. Simone Roach

2.   Nursing Diagnosis: An Obstacle of Caring Ways   11
    Gail Mitchell

3.   Technology and Caring in Nursing   24
    Rozzano C. Locsin

4.   Windows of Opportunity: Caring in Changing
    Political Climates   37
    Carol Picard and Galina Perfiljeva

5.   The Power of Caring: Issues and Strategies   48
    Madeleine Leininger

Part II   Power, Politics, and Public Policy: The Practice Lens   61

6. Unleashing the Giant: The Politics of Women's Health Care   63
    A. Lynne Wagner

7. Caring at the Crossroads: The Need for an Interpretive Strategy   82
    Patricia Farrell and Gary Nuttall

8. Values, Vision, and Action: Creating a Care-Focused Nursing
    Practice Environment   99
    Kathleen L. Valentine, Marilyn K. Stiles, and Deborah B. Mangan

9. Patients' Opinions of Mental Health Services in Russia   116
    Andrew Sosnovsky and Kathleen Valentine

10. Development of an Instrument to Assess Perceptions of Nurse
    Caring Behaviors Toward Family Members   131
    Lucie Gagnon and Sister Barbara Anne Gooding

11. A Nurse Leader's Dilemma: To Care or Not to Care   146
    Sandra S. Sweeney and Barbara A. Thomas

Part III   Power, Politics, and Public Policy: The Education Lens   157

12. The Curriculum Revolution in Nursing Education:
    The Caring Perspective and Its Relationship to Power,
    Politics, and Public Policy   159
    Roxie Thompson Isherwood

13. Professional Nurse Caring: Surviving the Transition
    to the Workplace   178
    Lesley M. Wilkes and Marianne C. Wallis

Preface

If we become capable of changing our vantage point, we possess a more varied perspective and thus free ourselves for more open thinking and for the higher stages of consciousness. (p. 22)

Hugo Enomiya-Lassalle
Living in the New Consciousness
(Boston: Sambhala
Publications, Inc., 1988)

Most chapters in this book represent scholarly papers presented at the 16th Caring Research Conference held in Ottawa, Canada, May 7–9, 1994, which was cohosted by the International Association for Human Caring, Inc. (IAHC). The central purpose of IAHC is to serve as a forum for all nurses, worldwide, who are interested in the advancement of the knowledge of human care and caring within the discipline of nursing.

The 1994 conference focused on power, politics, and public policy and how they relate to caring. *Power, politics,* and *public policy* connote a sense of distance, remoteness, and detachment. At first glance, these concepts may even appear antithetical to caring. A closer study, however, reveals the importance of interweaving caring into the fabric of society. Societal crises experienced today are indicative of a search for meaning in living. These crises point to the importance of reevaluating those values which guide actions.

Papers presented at this conference provide an impetus to reflect on the values that influence attitudes, views, and actions in relation to power, politics, and public policy. The organization of papers presents three different views: theory, practice, and education. Although the overall theme of each section may lead to a sense of commonality, each paper is unique and provides a particular perspective on the theme. It is hoped that this book will reinforce the commitment to caring that needs to direct our ways of being in the world. If caring can become the vantage point for our understanding of power, politics, and public policy, then these forces can be used to enhance the well-being of individuals and communities throughout the world.

I would like to express my gratitude to my coeditor, Kathleen Valentine, and to the authors and peer reviewers for their excellence in scholarship and their continued commitment to the goals of IAHC. The Board of IAHC warmly thanks its cosponsor, The Grey Bruce Regional Health Centre, of Ottawa, Canada, for making this special conference possible. We gratefully acknowledge the contributions and considerations of the Canadian Hospital Association and the Catholic Health Association of Canada. I also extend my appreciation to the readers and attendees of these conferences for your wonderful support. To Allan Graubard, Director of NLN Press, thank you for your continuing encouragement, commitment, and expertise.

Anne Boykin
President, IAHC

Peer Reviewers

Joyceen S. Boyle, PhD, RN
Professor and Chair
Department of Community Nursing
Medical College of Georgia
Augusta, GA

Nancy Case, PhD, RN
Undergraduate Program Director
Regis College
School of Nursing
Englewood, CO

Linda Dietrich, MS, RN
Director of Professional Practice
Kaiser Sunnyside Medical Center
Portland, OR

Delores Gaut, PhD, RN
Beaverton, OR

Cheryl Demerath Learn, PhD, RN
Lecturer
University of New Mexico
College of Nursing
Albuquerque, NM

Madeleine Leininger, PhD, RN,
FAAN
Professor
Wayne State University
College of Nursing
Detroit, MI

Ruth M. Neil, PhD, RN
Assistant Professor
University of Colorado
School of Nursing
Denver, CO

Marilyn E. Parker, PhD, RN
Florida Atlantic University
College of Nursing
Boca Raton, FL

Carol Picard, RNC, MS
Fitchburg State College
Fitchburg, MA

Barbara Place, PhD, RN
Ballarat University
School of Nursing
Ballarat, Victoria
Australia

Marilyn Ray, PhD, RN
Florida Atlantic University
College of Nursing
Boca Raton, FL

Sr. M. Simone Roach, PhD, RN
St. Augustine's Seminary
Scarborough, Ontario
Canada

Gwen Sherwood, PhD, RN
Assistant Dean for Educational
Outreach
University of Texas—Houston
School of Nursing
Houston, TX

Kathleen L. Valentine, PhD, RN
Director of Evaluation
University of Wisconsin
Eau Claire, WI

Robin J. Watts, PhD, RN
Head, School of Nursing
Curtin University of Technology
Pert, WA
Australia

Zane Wolfe, PhD, RN
Associate Professor
LaSalle University
School of Nursing
Ardmore, PA

Contributors

Anne Boykin, PhD, RN
Dean and Professor
College of Nursing
Florida Atlantic University
Boca Raton, FL

Patricia Lenore Farrell, MSc(A), BN,
RN, Doctoral Candidate
Associate Professor
Faculty of Nursing
University of Manitoba
Winnipeg, Manitoba, Canada

Lucie Gagnon, MSc, RN
Chargée D'Engeignement
Faculty of Nursing
University of Montreal
Montreal, Canada

Sister Barbara Anne Gooding, PhD,
RN
Associate Professor
School of Nursing
McGill University
Montreal, Canada

Roxie Thompson Isherwood, PhD, RN
Assistant Professor
Faculty of Nursing
The University of Calgary
Calgary, Alberta, Canada

Madeleine Leininger, PhD, RN,
FAAN
Professor
Wayne State University
College of Nursing
Detroit, MI

Rozzano C. Locsin, PhD, RNC
Assistant Professor of Nursing
Florida Atlantic University
College of Nursing
Boca Raton, FL

Malcolm R. MacDonald, EdD,
MScN, RN
Vice President Patient Care Services
The Grey Bruce Regional Health
Centre
Ontario, Canada

Deborah B. Mangan, MS, RN
Clinical Nurse Specialist
Department of Nursing
Mayo Clinic/Mayo Foundation
Rochester, MN

Gail Mitchell, PhD, RN
Chief Nursing Officer/Assistant
Professor
Sunnybrook Health Science Centre/
University of Toronto
North York, Ontario, Canada

Gary Nuttall, PEng, MA
Associate Professor
Faculty of Management
University of Manitoba
Winnipeg, Manitoba, Canada

Dr. Galina Perfiljeva
Dean, Faculty of Higher Nursing
Education
Moscow Medical Academy
Moscow, Russia

Carol Picard, MS, RNC
Assistant Professor
Fitchburg State College
Fitchburg, MA

Tim Porter-O'Grady, EdD, RN,
FAAN
Senior Partner, Tim Porter O'Grady
Inc.
Atlanta, GA

Sister M. Simone Roach, PhD, RN
St. Augustine's Seminary
Scarborough, Ontario, Canada

Andrew Sosnovsky, MD
The National Mental Health
Research Center
The Russian Academy of Medical
Sciences
Moscow, Russia

Marilyn Stiles, PhD, RN
Associate Consultant
Director of Nursing Research
Department of Nursing
Mayo Clinic/Mayo Foundation
Rochester, MN

Sandra Sweeney, PhD, RN
Professor
Department of Nursing Systems
University of Wisconsin—Eau Claire
Eau Claire, WI

Barbara Thomas, RN, MSN student
University of Wisconsin—Eau Claire
Eau Claire, WI

A. Lynne Wagner, MSN, FNP, RN
Associate Professor of Nursing
Fitchburg State College
Fitchburg, MA

M. C. Wallis, RN, PhD Candidate
Lecturer
Australian Catholic University
Sydney, New South Wales, Australia

L. M. Wilkes, PhD, RN
Associate Professor and Head of
School of Nursing and Human
Movement
Australian Catholic University
Sydney, New South Wales, Australia

Kathleen L. Valentine, PhD, RN
Assistant Professor
Director of Evaluation
Department of Nursing Systems
University of Wisconsin—Eau Claire
Eau Claire, WI

Introduction

Tim Porter-O'Grady

As the world changes at a rate faster than any of us can cope with, the challenges it presents are almost overwhelming. In every sector of our world the lives of men and women have been affected.

Driven by technological forces, of which we are as much the masters as the victims, our very experiences of life and our ways of knowing and acting must, it seems, keep apace. Since the introduction of the computer chip, a way of life is passing and being replaced by one that many of us have neither sought nor anticipated.

None of us is exempt from the implications of technology. In some way, every aspect of modern life is influenced or affected thereby. From telephones to toasters, the computer chip is imbedded in the tools of modern living. But something more is affected by the forces behind the technological winds of change. Our human experience, our way of knowing and relating to each other, is dramatically affected by the intrusion and action of technology on our culture and in our lives.

In the late 1960s and early 1970s, Marshall McLuhan gave warning that technology would one day make strangers of neighbors and neighbors of strangers. Television and satellite technology now can share the events halfway around the globe at the very minute they occur. Yet, at the same time, people seem totally unconnected to their next-door neighbors; indeed, they may not even know who they are. Who is neighbor? Who is stranger?

Inherently insulating and isolating, technology allows people to descend into their own reality; they can create their reality in a way that separates them from others and weakens the bonds of community. The relationships and interactions necessary to maintain community are negatively affected. Alienation, aloneness, nonidentification with others—all result in a social trauma whose extent has yet to be chartered. At the same time, our society seems little prepared to confront the realities accompanying the change.

Technology also allows us to do wonderful things. The very computer on which these words take their form allows the writer to connect to home base at will, to leave messages and to pick them up, to have conversations with people around the globe, to access every library database in the world, and to join the dialog on the Internet with a message and a viewpoint about any subject known to humankind. In regard to illness, technology is making the process of treatment easier and more portable, reducing the experiences of pain, suffering, separation from loved ones, and institutionalization for sickness. It is helping us all live longer and better without increasing the physical pain of the journey.

As we all sort through the impact of this transformation on our lives and our relationships, a tension continues between what is perceived as good about the emerging paradigm and what is clearly challenging. There is also hope, a possibility for new meaning, that may have tremendous implications and applications for the citizens of the world.

Technology is addressing much of what we once had to struggle to do and be: connect with each other, have dialogue from afar, monitor whole societies and mediate their conflicts, intervene in advance of or in response to cataclysmic events, avoid the trauma of war, violence, and other social or environmental grievances. We have tools to learn of our interdependence, the finiteness of our resources, and the fragility of life in all its forms. In fact, technology has helped us to understand interdependence as a truth of our life and has revealed its elegance and evils. We begin to comprehend the magnitude of all that can possibly be known and the fact that each of us can access that knowledge at any time we choose.

This new reality calls us to a deeper dialogue with and about each other. Just as technology has made us aware of our isolation and insulation, so too does it reveal our connectedness and all the variables that affect it. But we must deepen our dialogue in order to touch each other's lives at the core. Only then will we finally dispense with paradigms devoted to the more superficial and functional and touch the places of meaning in our lives, the connections that bind us together in our diverse richness and vulnerability.

We can and must stop actions that indicate that we are not yet connected to every piece of the fabric of civilization. Our vision of joy or suffering in the circumstance of a mother and her child must look the same in Africa as it does in America. Our response to tragedy and loss must show the same sympathy to pain in China as in Italy. We are capable of seeing the universal and we can no longer deny its presence. The only question that remains involves our response to what we see and know to be true.

In essence, technology is removing the barriers and walls that have kept us from truly seeing each other and bearing witness to the need for healing, caring, and connection. We can identify the global call for response to basic human needs, suffering, separation, evil, oppression, and maldistributed resources. We can testify to the injustice of wealth in resources, to the fruitfulness of one region of the earth and the arid emptiness of another. We are free to focus on our human relationships and the connections that make us a human community. The danger, however, is that we may get lost on the information highway and see technology as an end in itself.

Human caring is always about connection. Connection requires *presence*—a personal investment, a commitment to engage, a willingness to encounter whatever the interaction brings—and *time*—allowing for the encounter to develop mutually and to yield what is essential in the interaction. Without presence and time, no relationship is possible. But there lies the problem.

Because of our busyness, our artificial intelligence, and our global communication, we are tempted to become coopted by the technology, which often creates aloneness and insulation from each other. We have to make a conscious effort toward affiliation and purposefully abandon our isolation in favor of meaningful linkages that contain a whole range of healing moments. Healing is imbedded in relationship; not to enter into it is to avoid the opportunity to heal and be healed.

Within the current health care system, and because of the struggles to reconfigure it financially and structurally, there is a strong danger of miring in the process and missing the point of it all: *renewal*. When the system becomes the focus of the redesign, and its *purpose* can get lost in the shuffle. Health care, when seen in a limited way, is a system composed of a series of linkages that have to be addressed; it lacks a framework within which healing processes occur. Its structure has not meaning; it is a shell within which real value is not enclosed. Without a healing consciousness, the conversation becomes one of payers, providers, managed lives, critical paths, clinical outcomes, and systems alliances. The notions of health, community, care, connection, presence, and person get buried in the language and the structure.

Healers and caregivers are advocates of healing and health. Only they, it seems, can engage system planners and purveyors, and require that they focus on the purpose and intent of health service. Those who live at the point of care have the greatest stake in how responsive the system is and how much it reflects those whom it is directed to serve.

Healing as a semantic is forever expressed in the words of health care. Today, there are few players in the system who would not reference healing as a consideration that idealizes the character of our motives and the purpose to which our system is directed. But language is not enough. Articulating the value of healing or even enumerating its characteristics does not create the milieu that results in a healing context. Healing is a human activity. It requires care, connection, and skill in identifying and cooperating with the generative forces within the character and soul of the individual. Through the convergence of such personal and relational forces, we touch the elements of real healing.

But health reform as we know it expresses to us a very real tragedy: the reduction of health care to functionalism in its rawest form. Much of the change is mechanistic: a clear understanding of what must occur if society is to be healthy is missing. Health requires an awareness of what creates and supports it. If health is to be achieved, we must transform our concept of what it is and how we are going to achieve it. Communities need a different set of relationships, activities, and interactions to achieve an outcome that remotely resembles health. Shifting the providers around like pieces on a chessboard and rearranging the mechanisms used to pay them will not create healthy communities. We need health systems that care enough about the communities of which they are a part to engage them in a dialogue, build essential relationships, and begin to construct a healthy community.

Institutions are not obliged to take on alone the task of building toward health. Health will be an outcome of an exchange between health system and community, a recognition that health also means ownership of and investment in one's own pursuit of life. Here, providers can share their wisdom and the tools that they manipulate so well to facilitate the creation of health. The healer facilitates the interaction that is necessary to naming and applying processes that address the health needs of a community.

Sensitivity to culture is also essential. A culture must be allowed to define health within the context of its own values and experiences and to use those tools as a template for building health on cultural foundations. Indeed, caring requires that the science of health be deeply imbedded in specific and unique customs, forging a union or partnership between cultural practices and clinical processes. They interact in a dynamic construct that accrues value to people as a byproduct of their relationship. The healer and the healed then become interchangeable; both benefit from the experience and both are enhanced in its expression.

Retooling the mechanicisms of health care does not create the context for health. Today, the challenge is to do battle with the structures that are gravitating about the financial value stream in a way that impedes connections that lead to real health outcomes. In the sole interest of power positioning and economic configuring, health systems take the chance of losing their souls. They keep their distance from the issues of violence, poverty, homelessness, disenfranchisement, and personal brokenness, which are the foundations of much illness. When unaddressed, these conditions eventually create a tremendous negative impact on the provision of health care services. Providers end up treating the members of an unhealthy society who are driven into sickness by their unrelenting and unaddressed circumstances.

No health system can be sustained if it acts at cross-purposes with its core. We must create a milieu where caring and healing connections make it possible to address health as first priority of the system. As we learn more about reengineering and redesign of health services, it is important to keep in mind that such processes cannot succeed if they do not clearly and adequately address real need. They will only treat symptoms and forever leave the root causes untended. Unless root causes are dealt with, they will permanently poison the totality of our culture.

The move toward managed care as a capitated financial model in first-world countries has much to recommend it and just as much to incite caution. The difference between possibility and constraint here is intent and approach. Imbedded in the approach are signs of concern for health. Designing a system that assists people to manage their health and their lives better does help focus on personal and social issues. In this case, the thrust of both quality and cost concerns converges toward a system with the potential to raise community consciousness and personal accountability, and to focus attention on those factors that either facilitate health or inhibit it. To do this well, however, requires a focus beyond the short-term rewards identified by margins and revenues. We must look at success over the long term and commit resources toward provision of health services to communities. We must join with them in a mutually beneficial effort to produce sustainable health at both personal and collective levels.

The processes of case management, continuum of care structures, linkage of clinical services, partnership with the providers, and development of life management all serve to provide a positive framework for the delivery of well-motivated and coherent health services. This means breaking out of institutional models of illness' service, demolishing the cultural barriers that the current system exemplifies, bringing service to people, and partnering the providers with each other and with patients. All these actions represent subsets of what is good about managed care.

There are other risks, however. Managed care can focus on not providing service for its fixed dollars but, instead, allowing access to only "the best" subscribers—those whose health needs are minimal. Managed care leaders can develop relationships selectively so that the disadvantaged, who might compromise resources and limit profitability, never find their way to the services that the system offers. In essence, this is an unaccountable but revenue-intensive system that never confronts the needs of communities and is content with the health of its bottom line. There is a price for this, for both payer and provider: the economies of scale do not serve them well over the long term. As we well know, people forgotten by the system also eventually get sick and make demands through the back doors of hospitals and health systems, through emergency rooms, and in critical events that simply can't be ignored. Because they were left out early in their life process, the disenfranchised now present at the highest intensity of care and cost. Then, everyone pays, no one is benefited, and system viability is compromised.

A caring and healing community understands this situation as untenable. And the future requires, even more, that we, as part of this community, look critically at what the health care system is becoming. People are also required to become active with providers in developing approaches and models that address the effectiveness and viability of the health services. Partnership is paramount, and a partnership operates beyond the historic partisanship between providers. The partners see health in its broadest form, inclusive of and addressing the needs of the society of which it is a part.

In essence, this is what healing is all about. It is foundational to the character and content of the society and the individuals within whom it is found. Healing and caring are both a personal and a societal commitment; they address both the singular and the social. They reflect the quality of the soul and the character of the relationship within and between people. Their presence is a sign of the caring community and is witnessed by the comprehensiveness of health care—how it reaches out to every citizen, confronts issues and illnesses directly, and responds with compassion and concern.

The transformations with which we began can indicate either a demise of meaning and social viability or an awakening toward a broader and deeper reality. In health care, the transformation serves as a clarion call to critically examine the relationship between the health of a society and the well-being of its members. The moment challenges us all to connect in an intense dialogue about what can and should be done in the name of health. The constructs of the system should be examined closely to determine their viability and efficacy in meeting a community's need for health as well as its responsibility in seeking it.

Healing and caring reach the depth of their meaning and value as a collective experience. When a community of people gather together to join their energies and address the intensities of the moment and the needs of their members, the results of real healing and caring emerge. As agents and advocates of healing and caring, we—caregivers, nurses—can never forget that when we neglect our foundations, our need for each other, our purpose to connect and advance relationship, we fail to build a healthy community. If the current energies at redesigning health care reflect these truths and the outcomes testify to a truly healing intent, we can be sure that the effort will bear the fruit of our commitment to enrich and advance our human relationships and the health of our society. And, after all, that is what health care is all about.

Caring Connections

Malcolm R. MacDonald

Young nurse—eager, enthusiastic and bright
Scientifically trained, a head nurses' delight
Competent, efficient, proficient, well-grounded
In principles, protocols, processes, propounded.
Care maps, care plans, no problem too great
Organized, punctual, never ever late.
His peers adored him, even doctors took note
Of his promise, potential, credentials denote.
A professional unfolding, moulding to plans
Of other's intentions and systems' demands.
Yet promises to self, to serve unrestricted
Was a deep conviction conventions conflicted
For as he practiced with skilled head and skilled hands
His heart grew troubled with all the demands
Of patients, of people, the nursing profession.
He searched his books for answers to lessons.
The stress and strain of his continual giving
Getting fewer rewards to brighten his living.
He fretted, he frenzied, he frittered his time
Searching his textbooks line by line.
But no answers appeared, no insight was gained
The books were unyielding, his body was drained.
His spirit dispirited, his social interactions
Increasingly restricted, no healthy distractions.
Young nurse suffered in silence, confused,
And wary of giving, his talents unused.

When into his pathway a mentor appeared
An old nurse, a wise nurse, destiny steered.
A model of wisdom, a teacher of caring
Connected with self and with others' sharing.
She felt his feelings and through them she knew
This young nurse's journey was troubled but true.
Life's dips and valleys are lessons defined
But your trip is your trip
And my trip is mine.
Sort out your feelings and connect with your Source
Let Inner Voice guide you—an undauntable force.
Through connecting with self you connect with others
All creation created as sisters and brothers.
Not care, not care, but caring you fear
Rejoin the loose strands of creation to see clear
Awakening awareness that always was there
Connecting you, me and Thee and transforming care.
Young nurse listened intently but cried
"But wise nurse you know I've surely tried
To be the best nurse that I really can
I gave and I gave and I ran and I ran
Just give me a protocol to direct my approach
To life, to nursing, to avoid reproach."
Her presence was peaceful, her patient kind
For she knew that through experience, he'd ultimately find
The peace of caring, the meaning of love
Transforming, connecting, rising above
The disappointments, the misery, the fears and the pain
To a newfound meaning—so she repeated again
Life's dips and valleys are lessons defined
But your trip is your trip
And my trip is mine.
Sort out your feelings and connect with your Source
Inner Voice will guide you, an undauntable force.
Through connecting with self you connect with others
All creation created as sisters and brothers.
Not care, not care, but caring you fear
Rejoin the loose strands of creation to see clear.
Awakening, awareness that always was there
Connecting you, me and Thee and transforming care.
What did she mean, that caring old nurse?

Her words working inward were almost a curse.
He struggled with self and Inner Voice too
Until awakening, reverence, insight grew.
He stopped in silence as Inner Voice said,
"Not care, not care, but caring you dread."
So he committed to self and then to others
Genuine nurse caring for sisters and brothers
Daring to care through actions he found
Life positive, awesome, and relationships bound
Himself to others for mutual healing
The mysteries of life through care revealing.
He balanced his science with the art of caring
Growing in wisdom, wonder, and caring. Sharing
Himself with others in such peaceful understanding
That the struggles of nursing are so very demanding
Yet placed in our pathway so that we can find
Caring connections—body, spirit, and mind.
Connecting Ultimate Consciousness, you, me and Thee
All is one, miraculously, we are We.
So young nurse practiced nurse caring anew
Way beyond the nice little things for people we do
Through caring connections he healed, instilled hope
Relieved suffering through presence, helped others cope
Therapeutically touching a conduit for healing
Through intimate compassion, life's meaning revealing
Awakening, awareness, that always was there
Connecting you, me and thee and transforming care.
Then into his pathway a young nurse arrived
Scientifically trained, a novice in caring, she denied
That the secret of care is found in caring.
She studied, she searched, she researched for meaning
In frustration, confusion, dissolution, she asked
Old nurse, wise nurse for counsel, at last,
With Madonna smile, caring shone from his face
Old nurse responded with kindness and grace
Life's dips and valleys are lessons defined
But your trip is your trip
And my trip is mine.
Sort out your feelings and connect with your Source
Inner Voice will guide you—an undauntable force.
Through connecting with self you connect with others

All creation created as sisters and brothers
Not care, not care, but caring you fear
Rejoin the loose strands of creation to see clear
Awakening, awareness, that always was there
Connecting you, me and Thee and transforming care.

Part I

Power, Politics, and Public Policy:
The Theory Lens

1

The Dominant Paradigm of
the Modern World

Sister M. Simone Roach

We are now in the postmodern age. Perhaps the most striking thing we can say about this period is that it is marked by a breakdown of optimism. This breakdown—indeed, this crisis—has been described as "being condemned to the anxious space between the no-longer and the not-yet" (Rowe, 1980, p. 13). It constitutes a human challenge within which we locate "our horizons of expectation" (Toulmin, 1990). What are the major elements of this crisis?

The "no-longer" element of our present crisis is modernity itself. The beginning of the modern world, dated roughly in the 16th century, marked a major turning point in European history. Its founders, Isaac Newton, the intellectual giant of modern science, and René Descartes, mathematician and philosopher, radically changed the way we think about nature and reality. The period that followed is commonly referred to as the "enlightenment."

The enlightenment marked the beginning of the new cultural view of the modern age. The enlightenment itself envisioned liberation on many levels, challenging the previous hierarchical and static order. The shapers of this trend were encouraged by a perceived ability of the new worldview to shatter all so-called superstition and ignorance (religious belief and ideology) by unleashing the light of human reason. Advances in moral, political, and social thought led to an optimism that cast aside all doubts about its ability to achieve its goals on earth and in historical time. The builders of the modern age were determined to rid themselves of myth: reason alone was supreme.

According to Holland (1987), the liberalism flowing from the enlightenment shattered the hierarchical order of the premodern age and maximized autonomy of parts, competitive economics, and free thought. Religion became privatized; science became the religion of the public realm. This new vision, which became the cultural foundation of industrial capitalism, liberal democracy, and liberal culture, focused on "progress as evolution, freedom as competition, and a dualism of private religiosity and public secularism" (Holland, 1987, p. 46). The root metaphor of the machine has dominated the thinking of the modern period. Soelle and Cloyes (1984) find an apt representation of this phenomenon via the metaphor of the treadmill.

Along with liberalism, scientific Marxism challenged the premodern view in a revolutionary break from the past, but it criticized liberalism for not going far enough. Scientific Marxism dissolved the secular/religious dualism of liberalism into total secularization. "Autonomous secular science, centered in the state, emerges as the modern religion" (Holland, 1987, p. 49). Reason replaced fatalistic hierarchical rule, and the State became the absolute expression of reason. The root metaphor of scientific Marxism was still the machine but a "cybernetic one guided by intelligence—first in the revolutionary intelligentsia, then elite state bureaucrats" (p. 50).

The modern world, from the 16th century on, ushered in an age of ever-expanding progress in science and technology. In many ways, we, in the 20th century, are the beneficiaries of this extraordinary development. But the downside of modern culture, with its focus exclusively on the role of human reason, and with its personal (mind/body) and state (secular/religious) dualisms, is this: it built a "powerful and destructive scientific cage for humanity and nature. Worse than pre-modern fate, this modern fate threatens to destroy the earth and all humanity" (Holland, 1987, p. 41). The root metaphor of the machine has become the destructive force of both humanity and nature; the modern cultural, secular paradigm has shut out the awe and overarching inspiration of religious mystery. Over the past four centuries, we have become victimized by a value system that perceives technology as the "privileged mode of action in society," believing that all our problems can be solved by a "value-free scientific inquiry and value-free technological and social engineering" (Baum, 1985, p. 10).

As Solzhenitsyn (1978) reminds us, however, both capitalism and Marxism suffered from the same disease—the negation of anything higher than the human creature, a loss of the transcendent, a denial of the spiritual life. And, focusing on the outcome of this purely sensate worldview, Sorokin (1942) describes a crisis resulting from the decline of the sensate culture itself. Sorokin elaborates on this crisis as being marked by:

> . . . an extraordinary explosion of wars, revolutions, anarchy, and bloodshed; by social, moral, economic, political, and intellectual chaos; by a resurgence of revolting cruelty and animality, and a temporary destruction of the great and small values of mankind; by misery and suffering on the part of millions— a convulsion far in excess of the chaos and disorganization of the ordinary crises. (p. 22)

This sensate society, Sorokin continues:

> . . . has prepared its own surrender to the rudest coercion. "Liberating" itself from God, from all absolutes and categoric moral imperatives, it has become the victim of undisguised physical coercion and fraud. Society has reached the nadir of moral degradation and is now paying the tragic price of its own folly. Its vaunted utilitarianism, practicality, and realistic expediency have turned into the most impractical and dis-utilitarian catastrophe. Nemesis has at last overtaken it. (pp. 163–64)

Gibson Winter (1981), an American social ethicist, refers to the 20th century as "heir to deadly perils flowing out of industrial and technological development" (p. ix). These include the exhaustion of fossil resources stored up for billions of years; an endangered biosphere; the extinction of many forms of life; and human life itself threatened with annihilation by means of its own tools.

Fritjof Capra (1982), referred to as a "physicist turned mystic," notes the characteristics of a modern crisis resulting from "trying to apply the concepts of an outdated worldview—the mechanistic worldview of Cartesian–Newtonian science—to a reality that can no longer be understood in terms of these concepts" (pp. 15–16). Referring to our globally interconnected world in the biological, psychological, and environmental sense, Capra also speaks of the need for a new paradigm, a perspective that the view of our world as machine is incapable of offering.

Of particular significance is the title of Capra's work: The Turning Point (1982). On many fronts, our postmodern society stands in protest against its mechanistic roots; the machine metaphor is no longer compatible with our view of ourselves and of the world. But questions remain. Do we understand, and have we come to grips with the foundation of our problems? Do we have the will and the tools required to make the appropriate paradigm shift? Before examining the shift made by the caring paradigm, a brief examination of the impact of the mechanistic paradigm on the health world itself is in order.

THE MECHANISTIC PARADIGM
AND OUR HEALTH WORLD

Techno-society, with its mechanistic approach to progress, has introduced a wide spectrum of ethical problems that were unfamiliar to professionals and laypersons even a few years ago. Control over procreation, manipulation of genes, and preoccupation with quality of life as the priority and right of the individual are only a few of the challenges that beg for an approach other than that provided by an exclusively mechanistic, techno-rational perspective. The impact of the machine metaphor on the understanding of human biology is a case in point. Hans Jonas (1974), a Jewish philosopher, shows, for example, how biological engineering has profoundly changed our understanding of engineering itself. In the technical sense, engineering is understood to mean designing and constructing material artifacts for human use. In the past, its concern has been with lifeless materials. The advent of biological engineering, notes Jonas, "signals a radical departure from this clear division, indeed a break of metaphysical importance: Man becomes the direct object as well as subject of the engineering art" (pp. 142–143). With human genetic engineering, the experiment is the real deed for which mechanical engineering has no analog. Biological engineering can have unpredictable and irrevocable consequences.

A Canadian Federal Royal Commission on New Reproductive Technologies, after four years of hearings and written submissions from individuals and groups across Canada, issued its 1993 report, *Proceed with Care*. A major issue, framed in a variety of ways and raised in the majority of submissions, was the question of whether women ought to be subjected to biological experimentation in the first place. This was more than a control question. It was a question in the nature of: Should it be done at all? Does this not reflect Jonas's concern?

Nonetheless, the technological imperative, asserting that if a technology is available it ought to be used, has dominated our ethical choices. The use of technology has become an everyday issue in treatment protocols for the care of persons with irreversible conditions and has seriously complicated care decisions made by patients, their caregivers, and their families. And the dualisms of the religious/secular, private/public, personal/community, which prevail in our moral–ethical consciousness, make neither holistic care nor human ethical choices easier. Added to this is an almost exclusive emphasis on absolute autonomy at the core of our professional ethos. This focus on autonomy represents a further expression of the machine metaphor, a "parts" mentality, casting the individual out of his or her communal context and areas of responsibility. But, as reflected in postmodern literature, a paradigm shift has begun to occur.

THE TURNING POINT

In his 1982 work, *The Turning Point*, Capra stipulates that "modern physics has transcended the mechanistic Cartesian view of the world and is leading us to a holistic and intrinsically dynamic conception of the universe" (p. 97). Yet, in many areas and specifically in relation to health, Capra notes that the sense of physical, psychological, spiritual integrity, the sense of balance, has been lost in our culture. Winter (1981) makes a similar observation: "Even the medical profession gradually came to understand the human organism as a machine, developing technologized medicine around this imagery" (p. 5).

But the protest, as it has come from the person on the street and the professional, levies against any confusion here. The mechanistic, techno-scientific values that have shaped modern society can no longer sustain a civilized human community. Experiencing a sense of helplessness, the present generation seeks hope. Reduced to functional bodies, human beings seek personal wholeness. Having been nourished by the religion of secular humanism, persons seek a holistic spirituality. As a human community, we search for meaning; we hunger for the transcendent.

THE CHALLENGE OF A NEW METAPHOR

Winter (1981), challenging the machine as root metaphor of modern culture, speaks of the artistic metaphor as alternative: the need to live by an artistic, relational paradigm, to make visible the invisible through artistic representation and a world at play. Winter discusses metaphors as ways of knowing that give understanding to our world. Metaphors organize knowledge in particular ways, and different metaphors present different worlds. A shift in metaphors, and in ways of knowing and organizing, according to Winter, may reveal new insights into the nature of life and possibilities of human dwelling. He speaks of metaphor as a "vehicle of transcendence and freedom" (p. 8). A new metaphor creates the possibility of freeing ourselves from the shackles of the technological cage.

Acknowledging the positive values of technology, Winter's thesis is that artistic process best provides the integration of the mechanistic and organic, and is a power of transcending and liberation for which this age yearns in its agony of self-destruction. As he states:

> The root metaphor of artistic process, then, holds some promise of transcending the incoherence and anarchy of the mechanistic age. Metaphors do not settle everything, but they are guides to the rich possibilities of life and nature. When the decay of mechanical determinations holds a people in bondage, as seems to be the case in the technological order, we depend upon such metaphoric power to open a horizon of possibilities, with a vision to judge and liberate our age. (p. 24)

The International Association for Human Caring and the nursing profession at large offer a life-giving alternative to the mechanistic paradigm. In response to a letter to Gibson Winter, which focused on how his ideas on the artistic metaphor reflected nursing's recovery of its traditional charism of human care, Winter noted that the "more creative, caring understanding of the human being radically shifts the paradigm" (personal communication, March 27, 1993). Nursing as art is conceived, taught, managed, and practiced within a relational paradigm. Its power is what Mary Jo Leddy (1994), in her reflections on a work of Hannah Arendt (1959), calls "the energy that arises in the interaction of people . . . in the in-between of human relationships." This is power that cannot be stored up somehow for future use; it is enacted at every moment. Power, according to Arendt, exists only in its actualization, and it is actualized only where thoughts, words, and deeds come together. Its exercise does not need a crowd. It is what can happen when two people are in dialogue.

The caring paradigm is, in itself, a source of power. This caring power is highlighted in Fox (1979) and in McNeill, Morrison, and Nouwen (1982) as uncontaminated power, the kind of power that is not diluted by competition, driven to prestige or possessions, or motivated only by the urge to get to the top of the pyramid. Service, within the context of the caring paradigm, demands a suspicion of the power that is a fatal blindness, that considers every technological possibility worth doing, every career goal worth striving for, even if it means displacing or excluding others with a violence that fails to recognize our connectedness. Caring power is in the connection; it is in the relationship, exposed in the relational reality.

This paradigm shift has already occurred in nursing. We need only recall the focus of past IAHC conferences to realize how caring as a central concept in nursing has influenced practice, education, research, and administration. The present task of nursing is to espouse, with art and creativity, the human challenge the caring paradigm continues to present to us.

Caring is the human mode of being. We care not because we are health professionals; we care because we are human. In a world, in a society where the technologization of the human enterprise in politics, economics, and, indeed, in health care, has been destructive to life and human values, our commitment to professionalize the human capacity to care is a sign of hope. In calling forth this capacity in ourselves and in others, we become fulfilled as human beings.

Need we remind ourselves that our society is impoverished, in crisis, because we have lost our true identity as human persons, as a human community; because we have lost our sense of the transcendent, our capacity for awe before the mystery of creation? Unless we can somehow recapture our human dignity, grounded in the knowledge that we are wonderfully made in God's image; unless we recover our identity within a web of connectedness with all of creation, neither we nor this magnificent planet can survive.

The caring, artistic paradigm is already deeply embedded in the human psyche; the caring metaphor is the most accurate descriptor of the human journey. Our challenge to the mechanistic paradigm, which has shaped power, politics, and public policy in Western society, is to retrieve human care, and to continue to make it more visible, not only within the health professions but within the whole of our society. Parochial professionalism will not do this. Our challenge is to be professionals who are first and foremost human citizens who know and live out the meaning of connectedness with each other and with all of creation.

Loren Eiseley (1960), an anthropologist, reminds us of the connection between care and human survival, of how the power of human care structured even the primitive way of life, of how politics and policy seemed to have responded to the unique contingencies of human living at that earlier period of time. His words provide a fitting conclusion to this chapter:

> Forty thousand years ago, in the bleak uplands of southwestern Asia, a man, a Neanderthal man, once labeled by the Darwinian proponents of struggle as a ferocious ancestral beast—a man whose face might cause you some slight uneasiness if he sat beside you—a man of this sort existed with a fearful body handicap in that ice-age world. He had lost an arm. But still he lived and was cared for. Somebody, some group of human things, in a hard, violent and stony world, loved this maimed creature enough to cherish him. (pp. 144–145)

REFERENCES

Arendt, H. (1959). *The human condition*. New York: Doubleday/Anchor Books.
Baum, G. (1985). Faith and culture. *The Ecumenist, 24,* 9–13.

Capra, F. (1982). *The turning point: Science, society and the rising culture.* Toronto: Bantam Books.

Eiseley, L. (1960). *The firmament of time.* New York: Atheneum.

Fox, M. (1979). *A spirituality named compassion.* Minneapolis: Winston Press.

Holland, J. (1987). The post-modern paradigm implicit in the church's shift to the left. In M. J. Leddy (Ed.), *The faith that transforms* (pp. 39–61). New York: Paulist Press.

Jonas, H. (1974). *Philosophical essays: From ancient creed to technological man.* Chicago: The University of Chicago Press (Midway Reprint).

Leddy, M. J. (1994, March). Women and redeeming power. *Catholic New Times,* pp. 10–11.

McNeill, D. P., Morrison, D. A., & Nouwen, H. J. M. (1982). *Compassion: A reflection on the Christian life.* New York: Doubleday.

Rowe, S. C. (1980). *Living beyond crisis: Essays on discovery and being in the world.* New York: Pilgrim Press.

Royal Commission on New Reproductive Technologies. (1993). *Proceed with care.* Ottawa: Minister of Government Services of Canada.

Soele, D. & Cloyes, S. A. (1984). *To work and to love.* Philadelphia: Fortress Press.

Solzhenitsyn, A. (1978). *A world split apart.* New York: Harper & Row.

Sorokin, P. (1942). *The crisis of our age.* New York: Dutton.

Toulmin, S. (1990). *Cosmopolis: The hidden agenda of modernity.* New York: Free Press.

Winter, G. (1981). *Liberating creation: Foundations of religious Social ethics.* New York: Crossroad.

2

Nursing Diagnosis:
An Obstacle of Caring Ways

Gail Mitchell

Nursing diagnosis, as a process of assessing, judging, and labeling, is an obstacle to caring ways. As a practice discipline, nursing's phenomena of concern involve human experiences of health. It must be emphasized that the diagnostic approach itself is being challenged here, and not merely a particular diagnostic framework, such as the taxonomy developed by the North American Nursing Diagnosis Association (NANDA). The process of nursing diagnosis engenders—indeed, necessitates—a particular attitude or approach, and it is this attitude that obstructs caring ways in practice. The possibility that the diagnostic approach obstructs caring ways is worthy of investigation because many nurses and their professional organizations advance the belief that the diagnostic process is an essential requirement of professional practice (Caroll-Johnson, 1988; Gordon, 1987; Harrington, 1988).

Before clarifying the issues surrounding diagnosis, I will briefly comment on my own views of nursing, health, and caring, so that others may more fully evaluate this critique. My practice and research activities are guided by the nursing theory called human becoming (Parse, 1981, 1987, 1992). This theory, crafted by Parse in 1981, focuses on the centrality of lived experience and the structure of meaning in relation to health and human becoming. The goal in practice is quality of life as defined by persons themselves (Parse, 1987,

1992). Nurses guided by Parse's theory live caring ways through true presence as persons disclose the meaning of health experiences while relating value priorities and moving toward personal hopes and dreams.

This chapter offers three basic assumptions about human beings that are essential to the caring process. The assumptions flow from the theoretical perspective of Parse's theory, which forms the foundation of the particular understanding of caring described below. The three requirements essential for caring ways are:

1. Caring ways require the theoretical assumption that human beings are complex beyond knowing.

2. Caring ways require the theoretical assumption that human beings are the inventive participants of health-related projects.

3. Caring ways require the theoretical assumption that human beings hold unbounded possibility.

Each of these statements can be discussed in light of the diagnostic attitude.

HUMAN BEINGS ARE COMPLEX BEYOND KNOWING

The first requirement of caring ways is a theoretical belief system that regards persons as *complex beyond knowing*. This means that a nurse will foster caring ways if the client is approached as an entity that is not knowable in a definitive or preestablished way. A nurse may learn something about another in the moments of a practice engagement. The complexity of the other's living may be glimpsed, but a nurse cannot know all that the person's lived experience encompasses. Life cannot be decomposed into parts or problems because it is a unity of interrelationships (Gadamer, 1989). Further, what can be known in any moment changes as persons disclose the multidimensional and paradoxical profiles symbolic of lived experience (Mitchell, 1993a; Moch, 1989; Parse, 1981, 1992).

Caring as an attitude or an action requires respect for the mystery that human beings are. Persons by their nature are continuously changing and becoming more diverse (Parse, 1981, 1992). To be caring, a nurse must be innocent and open when approaching another—not innocent in an unknowing way, but innocent in a nonjudging, nonassuming way. Any system of thought that attempts to predefine human experience based on an expert's knowing is restrictive in the extreme and inherently obstructive to caring ways. In addition, the discomfiting consequences for nurses who are educated to see clients as the sum of their problems and diagnoses have yet to be explicated. The diagnostic attitude exerts a silent but taxing burden for some nurses who are asked to judge, label, and fix other human beings. This burden is consistent with Covey's (1989) insight that it is "much more ennobling to the human spirit to let people judge themselves, than to judge them" (p. 224).

An assumption of the diagnostic approach is that the expert does know, or can come to know in some definitive and prescriptive way. Carpenito (1983) claims that the nurse can define and order the *definitive* interventions that control and manage the health of another. Some authors claim that a taxonomy of diagnoses will allow nurses to label clients' conditions consistently through generalizations based on the assessment of common problems and standardized outcomes (Anderson & Briggs, 1988; Aydelotte & Peterson, 1987; Burns, 1991; Maas & Hardy, 1988).

Assessment protocols and tools consistent with the diagnostic approach extract bits of information from the unitary nexus of the person's lived experience. This information is then viewed as objective and comparable to standards of normality (Maas & Hardy, 1988). Even if the assessment protocol is acknowledged as not yet adequate, the grounding assumption of diagnosis is that, with more research and further application and testing, the knowledge of human experience will be verified. Derdiarian (1988) proposed that "research should determine, describe, and validate nursing diagnoses as well as their manifestations in verifiable indicators and causes" (p. 139). The search for verifiable indicators is rooted in the experts' belief that human beings can be known with some degree of certainty. Bruss (1988) attempted to verify the diagnosis of hopelessness using a predefined list of criteria. The criteria included acontextual bits of information such as sighing, decreased appetite, shrugging, turning away from the speaker, and closing eyes (Bruss, 1988).

It is interesting to note that some of these same actions were disclosed by people describing their discomfort with the diagnostic attitude of nurses (Mitchell, 1991). Persons who believed that nurses were judging them and showing disregard for their unique situations also turned away, became silent, and closed their eyes. An infinite number of theoretical explanations can be offered for actions observed in practice. The diagnostic process assumes and seeks to discover an objective reality that few scholars now endorse, given the present understanding of knowledge development (Bernstein, 1988; Gadamer, 1989; Heidegger, 1962).

What exactly do the experts verify when they identify generalizable indicators? It has been proposed that what a professional reveals when assessing and diagnosing a client is not what is present in the client's reality, but, rather, the professional reveals what is within his or her own reality (Covey, 1989). This statement prompts a pause. If we think about the "professional" assessment, and picture a team of experts sitting around a table discussing various interpretations and diagnoses that summarize the client's situation, the meaning of the statement becomes dramatically evident. The expert team reveals their own theoretical knowledge, their values and beliefs about who the person is, and their opinions about who the person can become. The expert finds his or her own knowing in the other; thus, the diagnostic process limits what another human being can be to what the expert knows. If the expert only knows deficits and dysfunctions, abnormalities and pathologies, inadequacies and alterations, then the knowing of the recipients of the expert's care will be restrictively predefined by these categories. Gadamer (1989) challenged the self-regarding nature of those who seek to predict the behaviors of other persons. He claimed it is simply a means to their own ends. In a similar light, Hagey and McDonough (1984) suggested that "either supporters of nursing diagnosis see the categories as harmless without social context or they take as self-evident and acceptable the political outcomes that such categories may produce" (p. 153). The outcomes of the diagnostic attitude include oppression and restriction for clients and nurses.

The diagnostic process is based on the belief that the expert knows about human health. This widely embraced assumption has serious implications. It is suggested here that nurses guided by the diagnostic approach disregard the person's unique experience of health because it is the problem that is prized and knowable. Problem identification and management are, after all, the desired outcomes of the diagnostic assessment and, once identified, the problem gets brought up close in a tunneling kind of way, and the person's life gets viewed through the expert's limited vision (Hagey & McDonough, 1984; McHugh, 1986; Shamansky & Yanni, 1983). This tunnel vision is not merely limited in scope but it may be argued that it is potentially harmful for recipients of care. Consider the following quote by Deegan (1993), who was describing the restrictions of having a diagnosis applied to her life:

> The professionals are telling you that you are a schizophrenic. Your family and friends are beginning to refer to you as a schizophrenic. It is as if the whole world has put on a pair of warped glasses that blind them to the person you are and leaves them seeing you as an illness. It seems that everything you do gets interpreted through the lenses of these warped glasses. If you don't laugh, that is worrisome and, if you laugh too much, that is also worrisome. If you don't move, they get alarmed and, if you move around too much, they get alarmed. The range of behaviors and feelings you are allowed has been dramatically narrowed as a result of the blinders that those around you have put on. (p. 14)

After patients are diagnosed as having a problem identified from the expert's frame of reference, they are subjected to ongoing surveillance. As Deegan reported, once the diagnosis is applied, all thoughts and actions expressed in the presence of others get interpreted as signs and symptoms of the problem or dys-function. The burden of this surveillance is harmful for various reasons, for ex-ample, the isolation of feeling misunderstood (Mitchell, 1994a). Interpretation and understanding are inseparable (Gadamer, 1989); thus, the nurse's under-standing of the other is also imprisoned in the diagnostic attitude. Scott-Maxwell (1968) wrote about a phenomenon she called false cheerfulness—a pretense that patients show to expert nurses so that they will not detect the struggles, angers, frustrations, and sorrows that are lived in the clients' reali-ties. Clients learn to protect and hide their precious realities from the critical eyes of the expert diagnosticians. A woman living in a chronic care setting re-ported that her pain and suffering happened in the dark of the night so that others would not know. She said her crying was silently lived and hidden from nurses who do not care.

Following diagnosis, persons are expected to follow treatments, to be com-pliant, and to live according to norms and rules that are also problem- and provider-focused. The writing of one older women who was hospitalized with a fractured hip captures the inherent harm of being judged and treated like a problem: "What if I became a burden, ceased to be a person and became a prob-lem, a patient. . . . That was my one fear. [So] I must conform. I must be correct. I must be meek, obedient, and grateful, on no account must I be surprising. If I deviate by the breadth of a toothbrush, I would be in the wrong" (Scott-Maxwell, 1968, p. 91). As long as the provider is the one who assumes to know the person, and the meaning of health and quality of life, caring ways will not be possible.

HUMAN BEINGS ARE INVENTIVE PARTICIPANTS

The second essential requirement for caring ways is *a theoretical belief system that assumes human beings are inventive participants in health-related projects.* Car-ing ways require that the *caregiver* see persons as the coauthors of their lives, the inventive originators of their health-related projects. Freedom is a basic tenet of human science (Dilthey, 1976, 1883/1988) and a specific value in many nurs-ing and organizational statements of philosophy. Yet, few would argue that the client's right to freely participate in care remains a distant ideal. A nurse can-not be caring if others are viewed as less than coparticipants in the living of their health. The others' own power of healing requires respect and nurturing. Nursing diagnosis obstructs caring ways because of disregard for the person's power and participation in living health and in creating desired change.

Although not acknowledged by all proponents of nursing diagnosis (New-man, 1986), it is proposed here that the traditional diagnostic attitude is underpinned by deterministic and mechanistic principles. Determinism proposes that human beings are controlled by probabilistic laws of human nature. Laws that are causal or probabilistic lead the expert to search for relevant variables in order to predict and control human responses to experiences like grieving a loss, struggling with change, or living with cancer or Alzheimer's disease. Behaviorism, an approach based on the principle of stimulus–response, continues to have a major influence in nursing. There is essentially no arena or opportunity for inventive participation in the stimulus–response interaction.

Diagnosis perpetuates the notion that complex life situations are reducible to actual or potential problems that should be fixed, eliminated, or managed by experts. This assumption ignores the inherent growth that comes from experience itself through the process of choosing one's way and having the freedom and dignity to make one's own mistakes. The goal of a practice based on the processes of assessing, judging, and labeling is to eliminate problems. What then happens to the universal experience of learning from life's mistakes (Mitchell, 1994b; Scott-Maxwell, 1968)? Many old people speak of learning from life's blunders and of becoming wise, fine, and supple from mistakes that refine an astuteness for guiding life choices (Mitchell, 1994; Scott-Maxwell, 1968).

Additionally, what happens to the unexpected benefits that come from what at first might seem to be undesirable situations? What does it mean when people say things like, "I am glad this happened even though it was terrible, because it gave me a chance to reexamine my life and to decide what is important for me." How is it that Mary Fischer (1994?), the author of *Sleep with the Angels,* refers to herself as inspired and blessed when to outsider experts she is judged to be a tragic victim, a young mother diagnosed with AIDS? As a nurse, I am left wondering what opportunities to contribute to health will continue to be smothered under the shroud of the diagnostic attitude.

Caring ways require an acknowledgment of the dignity of risk (Deegan, 1993) and a valuing for the making of one's own mistakes. Nurses cannot truly live caring ways in practice if they are unwilling to consider not only persons' right to live with risk, but also the right to decide which risks are worth taking. For example, an elderly man, Mr. R, was admitted to an acute care setting in order to be assessed for a gait disturbance following several falls over a period of three weeks. None of the falls resulted in serious injury, but the multidisciplinary team, armed with the diagnoses of impaired gait and ineffective coping, decided he was too much at risk to return home safely.

Mr. R, on the other hand, said that he knew he might fall, but he also knew he wanted to live that risk because to go to a nursing home was impossible. He said he would sooner die than not be able to have his own place. He told a nurse that he had worked things out, that he knew how to fall so he would not hurt himself. The nurse in this situation, guided by Parse's theory, was open and respectful of his perspective and his right to choose which risks were worth taking in life. The nurse's openness to Mr. R's wishes and concerns, and to his right to choose and participate in life, demonstrates caring ways.

The notion of protecting old people from risk is often rooted in an unexamined prejudice. Who would tell a young person that he or she should not go skying because a fall might happen? Young people choose the risks they want to live with—most people do; but health care professionals have trouble honoring the same choice of risk among older people or people judged to be ill.

In contrast to the belief that human beings are controlled by deterministic laws is the belief that human beings participate in making life what it is, based on their choosing from options encountered in daily life. Parse's (1981) nursing theory is rooted in the existential tenet of *situated freedom:* human beings in every situation are faced with choices about how to proceed, what to think, whom to relate with, what attitude to have, what dreams to imagine, and what meaning to give to different happenings. Some nurses contend that the poor, the disadvantaged, and the disabled do not make choices in life. These nurses obviously believe that human choice is linked to economics, genetics, and social strata. But situated freedom considers the dignity of choice to be an inherent quality of human life. Whether imprisoned (Frankl, 1959), or living in the slums of Calcutta (Lapierre, 1991), or living with quadriplegia or Alzheimer's disease in a chronic care institution (Mitchell, 1993b), human beings make choices about how to be and how to look at their situations, and they undoubtedly ponder what is important to quality of life. Caring in the nurse–person relationship must be redirected to attend to human freedom and the invention of health experiences.

A young man offered the following description about choice and health:

You see I am a quadriplegic, that is what I live with, it is part of who I am. But day to day I do not think about being paralyzed. I think about living and reaching my goals, and working things out, getting what I need, just like you do. And some of the obstacles I face are created by me. I can choose how do I want to think about this or that. I could be angry, but I'm not angry because I'm too concerned about who I can be, given the things I live with. Anger can help me express who I am and it helps me to go on. I have lots of strategies for living and for keeping quality in my life. (Mitchell, 1993b)

HUMAN BEINGS POSSESS
UNBOUNDED POSSIBILITY

The third essential requirement for caring ways is a theoretical assumption that *persons hold unbounded possibility.* Only a theoretical view that is open to persons' inherent potential to go beyond, to become more, and to exceed expectations, will nurture caring ways. If nurses are open to persons' unbounded possibilities, then they will also be open to learning how people integrate change while creating health. Strasser (1967) points out that a person's unique possibilities relate to the belief that a human being is always more than he or she seems, because designs for change are already present in the person's anticipation of the not-yet. Similarly, Heidegger (1962) proposed that the human being has already chosen certain possibilities and is always projecting toward others, in the throwness and facticity of life. He said that persons know and understand what possibles are possible for their ownmost potentiality-for-Being. To live caring ways in practice, the nurse must see the person as the discloser of possibilities rather than the unknowing receiver of possibles defined by experts.

A nurse cannot truly care for others when a ceiling has already been placed on who the person can be and become. The attitude perpetuated by the diagnostic process can only be called an attitude of arrogance. That an expert could assume to know what another should think or do following an assessment process insults the very dignity of what it is to be human, in all its wonder and complexity. Nurses who approach others with the expectation that they should be "normal" limit what can happen in the nurse–person relationship.

The whole concept of normality is antithetical to change and uniqueness, two concepts essential to human life. There is no blueprint for how people should live or experience health. There is no best way to grieve, to cope, to love, or to despair. Rather than identifying diagnoses according to the expert's frame of reference, nurses could choose to learn about how human beings integrate change, how they invent strategies for living on, what people learn from mistakes, and how persons think about and shift value priorities for creating health and quality of life.

Even though the expert is guided to ask the person's perspective in some diagnostic assessments (Gordon, 1987), the individual's view is often judged as appropriate-or-not, realistic-or-not, cooperative-or-not—according to the expert's assessment of the situation. The medicalization of the person and the life process has been thoroughly and diligently executed. Fortunately, human beings continue to choose their own way despite the directives of experts. A psychologist shared the following insight about expert advice: "Today I recalled the difficulty always experienced in making people do what it is they ought to do, even with the most severe methods tried, and . . . my hopes rose a little" (Scott-Maxwell, 1968, p. 135).

Human beings do not view their lives through diagnostic labels. Rather, they integrate changes, concerns, illnesses, losses, and unexpected events into a life that is already being lived, a life that is unitary in nature and that is beyond the expert's knowing. Research on quality of life from the client's perspective surfaced awareness about the opportunities nurses have to influence quality of life (Mitchell, 1993b). Young people living with quadriplegia and multiple sclerosis, and older people living with Alzheimer's disease, spoke of the importance of relationships for quality of life. If these people had said that the quality of their lives was defined by their disabilities and illnesses, there might be less hope, and less opportunity for making a difference. But to know that quality of life relates to things like the ways nurses are with clients and the ways nurses speak, and touch, and care—this means nurses could expand practice to new realms of participating with the inventiveness of the human health experience.

Unfortunately, the ways people integrate changes in life have not been viewed by nurses as the foundation for a practice aimed at changing health and quality of life. Nurses need to begin to learn from people, so that enhanced understanding and knowledge of how health is experienced in the midst of illness, struggle, joy, disability, loss, and pain can be developed. The meaning of lived experiences is beyond the knowledge of the outsider. As aptly noted by Florida Scott-Maxwell, "I observe others, but I experience myself. Who could be as helpful to me as myself, muddled creature that I am, since it is my mortification, my respect that tells me what is real" (1968, p. 19).

COMPARING PRACTICE APPROACHES

A basic assumption of this chapter is that the knowledge of the nurse guides actions and attitudes in practice. To help demonstrate this claim, a situation from practice is presented here from two perspectives. The first view was compiled by a nurse who was guided by the traditional nursing process with diagnosis.

Jim, a man living with AIDS, was admitted for what would be his last time; he was diagnosed as having pneumonia. He frequently spoke to nurses of his plans to get out of the hospital and to go to the mountains or to the beach. Nurses were concerned because they believed Jim's death was imminent and they knew he would not get out of the hospital. The nurses thought Jim's dreams were unrealistic, and two new diagnoses were added to his care plan: "dysfunctional grieving" and "ineffective coping." These guided nurses to try to get Jim to accept his impending death, and various measures were introduced to improve his coping skills. Each day, if Jim talked about his dreams to get out of the hospital, nurses tried to divert his thoughts. A consult to pastoral services was initiated to help him grieve and cope with death.

Now consider a different view of the same man, when the person is assumed to be complex beyond knowing, an active participant in health, and the holder of unbounded possibility. The nurse in this later situation was guided by Parse's

(1981, 1987, 1992) theory of human becoming. Jim says that life is getting more and more difficult. One thing that helps him to get through the day is his thoughts of what he would love to be doing. Pretending that everything is OK and that he will go to the mountains one day gives Jim a boost. Pretending to be somewhere else helps Jim to move away from the pain of his situation for a little while. He knows that he wants to live, and yet he wants to die and move on. Jim plans to go to the beach one more time, even if he makes it only in his dreams.

The nurse, guided by Parse's theory, did not judge or diagnose the way Jim was living his dying. She did not approach him with an attitude that conveyed a message that she was the expert about his life, health, and impending death. In seeing him as an inventive participant in his health, the nurse centered discussion on ways Jim helped himself to go on, and they talked about what it was like in the mountains and on the beach. Picturing how things could be is also a way of being there and of transcending difficult situations (Parse, 1981, 1992). By being a holder of possibilities, Jim creates the meanings, dreams, and hopes that shape his health, his death, and the quality of his life. Pretending is a way of moving beyond; it is one of many possibilities that Jim created as an inventive participant in health.

MOVING BEYOND THE DIAGNOSTIC ATTITUDE

If experts reveal themselves in what they speak, and in how they know and view clients, then nurses may want to consider what they *want* to see, how they *want* to think of persons, and what they *want* to value in their relationships with others. There are no limits on the number of theoretical interpretations that can provide explanations for understanding human health experiences. Perhaps it is, frankly, a matter of choice, a choosing of values that upholds a professional commitment to caring ways. There is compelling evidence to support the notion that all science boils down to values—to choice, deliberation, and commitment (Bernstein, 1988; Kaplan, 1974). And, as noted noted by Guba and Lincoln (1990), there is no support for objective, value-free knowledge of any sort. This value-ladenness is precisely why nurses require theoretical belief systems that nurture and are consistent with caring ways in practice and research.

Nursing diagnosis has been challenged in the literature by relatively few nurses (Hagey & McDonough, 1984; McHugh, 1986; Mitchell, 1991; Mitchell & Santopinto, 1988; Shamansky & Yanni, 1983), and it continues to be promoted without question and integrated into standards of practice. Many professional associations throughout North America define nursing according to the diagnostic process. The purpose of this chapter is to provoke thinking about diagnosis as an obstacle to caring ways. It is my hope that the assumptions underpinning both diagnosis and caring will be further explored and that nurses will continue to question and debate the assumptions and outcomes of all practice approaches, so that choices can reflect the commitment and choice to serve people and promote health. Gadamer (1989) suggests that practice is a presentation of self, and that the language of a science is symbolic of an expressive field of the members who are the discipline. Nurses could choose an expressive field that honors and values human mystery, inventiveness, and potentiality for being. Not every field nurtures caring ways. In order to nurture caring ways, nurses must define their expressive fields of knowledge in nursing theories that uphold essential values about human beings and their living of health.

REFERENCES

Anderson, J. E., & Briggs, L. L. (1988). Nursing diagnosis: A study of quality and supportive evidence. Image: The Journal of Nursing Scholarship, 20(3), 141–144.

Aydelotte, M. K., & Peterson, K. H. (1987). Keynote address: Nursing taxonomies—state of the art. In A. M. Mclane (Ed.), Classification of nursing diagnoses—Proceedings of the Seventh Conference (pp. 1–16). St. Louis: Mosby.

Bernstein, R. J. (1988). Beyond objectivism and relativism: Science, hermeneutics, and praxis. Philadelphia: University of Pennsylvania Press.

Bruss, C. R. (1988). Nursing diagnosis of hopelessness. Journal of Psychosocial Nursing and Mental Health Services, 26(3), 28–31.

Burns, C. (1991). Develop and content validity testing if a comprehensive classification of diagnosis for pediatric nurse practitioner. Nursing Diagnosis, 2(3), 93–104.

Caroll-Johnson, K. M. (Ed.). (1988). Classification of nursing diagnosis: Proceedings of the Eighth Conference. Philadelphia: Lippincott.

Carpenito, L. J. (1983). Nursing diagnosis: Application to clinical practice. Philadelphia: Lippincott.

Covey, S. R. (1989). The 7 habits of highly effective people. New York: Simon & Schuster.

Deegan, P. E. (1993). Recovering our sense of value after being labeled. Journal of Psychosocial Nursing, 31(4), 7–11.

Derdiarian, A. (1988). A valid profession needs valid diagnosis. Nursing & Health Care, 9, 137–140.

Dilthey, W. (1976). *Selected writings* (H. P. Rickman, Trans.). Cambridge, England: Cambridge University Press.

Dilthey, W. (1988). *Introduction to the human sciences* (R. J. Bentanzo, Trans.). Detroit: Wayne State University Press. (Original work published 1883.)

Fischer, M. (1994). *Sleep with the angels.* Wakefield, RI: Mayer Bell.

Frankl, V. (1959). *Man's search for meaning: An introduction to logotherapy* (I. Lasch, Trans.). Boston: Beacon Press.

Gadamer, H.-G. (1989). *Truth and method* (2nd ed.). (J. Weinsheimer & D. G. Marshall, Trans.). New York: Crossroad.

Gordon, M. (1987). *Nursing diagnosis process and application* (2nd ed.). New York: McGraw-Hill.

Guba, E. G., & Lincoln, Y. S. (1990). Can there be a human science? Constructivism as an alternative. *Person-Centered Review, 5*(2), 130–154.

Hagey, R. S., & McDonough, P. (1984). The problem of professional labeling. *Nursing Outlook, 32,* 151–157.

Harrington, L. (1988). The diagnosis dilemma: One preferred remedy. *Nursing & Health Care, 9,* 93–94.

Heidegger, M. (1962). *Being and time* (J. Macquarrie & E. Robinson, Trans.). New York: Harper & Row.

Kaplan, A. (1974). Values in inquiry. In G. Riley (Ed.), *Values, objectivity and the social sciences* (pp. 84–101). Reading, MA: Addison-Wesley.

Lapierre, D. (1991). *The city of joy.* New York: Warner Books.

Maas, M., & Hardy, M. (1988). Focus: Nursing diagnosis—Challenge for the future. *Journal of Gerontological Nursing, 14*(3), 8–13.

McHugh, M. K. (1986). Nursing process: Musings on the method. *Holistic Nursing Practice, 1*(1), 21–28.

Mitchell, G. J. (1991). Nursing diagnosis: An ethical analysis. *Image: The Journal of Nursing Scholarship, 23*(2), 99–103.

Mitchell, G. J. (1993a). Living paradox in Parse's theory. *Nursing Science Quarterly, 6,* 44–51.

Mitchell, G. J. (1993b, November). *Quality of life: The client's perspective.* Paper presented at The Queen Elizabeth Hospital, Toronto, Ontario.

Mitchell, G. J. (1994a, January 28). *Quality of life for persons living with Alzheimer's disease.* Paper presented at the 7th Annual Alzheimer's Symposium, Mount Sinai Medical Center, Toronto, Ontario.

Mitchell, G. J. (1994b). The meaning of being a senior. *Nursing Science Quarterly, 7,* 70–79.

Mitchell, G. J., & Santopinto, M. D. A. (1988). An alternative to nursing diagnosis. *The Canadian Nurse, 84*(10), 25–28.

Moch, S. D. (1989). Health within illness: Conceptual evolution and practice possibilities. *Advances in Nursing Science, 11*(4), 23–31.

Newman, M. (1986). Nursing's emerging paradigm: The diagnosis of pattern. In A. M. McLane (Ed.), *Classification of nursing diagnosis: Proceedings of the Seventh Conference*. St. Louis: Mosby.

Parse, R. R. (1981). *Man-living-health: A theory of nursing*. New York: Wiley.

Parse, R. R. (1987). *Nursing science: Major paradigms, theories, and critiques*. Philadelphia: Saunders.

Parse, R. R. (1992). Human becoming: Parse's theory of nursing. *Nursing Science Quarterly, 5*, 35–42.

Scott-Maxwell, F. (1968). *The measure of my days*. New York: Penguin.

Shamansky, S. L., & Yanni, C. R. (1983). In opposition to nursing diagnosis: A minority opinion. *Image: The Journal of Nursing Scholarship, 15*, 47–50.

Strasser, S. (1967). Phenomenologies and psychologies. In N. Lawrence & D. O'Connor (Eds.), *Readings in existential phenomenology* (pp. 331–351). Englewood Cliffs, NJ: Prentice-Hall.

3

Technology and Caring in Nursing

Rozzano C. Locsin

In the November–December 1993 issue of *The American Nurse,* the official newspaper of the American Nurses Association, two articles (Casetta, 1993a; Casetta, 1993b) describe the prominence that technology has attained in contemporary nursing practice. These articles describe the evolution and definition of "high-tech" nursing as essentially caring for technology-dependent patients who require intensive support in specialized units. High-tech nurses are achievement-oriented practitioners who have a level of competence that complies with the advanced nature of technology, which allows them a more expeditious way of processing interventions for technology-dependent patients.

Ethical decisions in high-tech nursing focus on issues about the quality of a patient's life with or without technological support. Nurses are in a position to make assessments about the best course of action for each individual because of the time they spend with patients. Some professional nurses are more comfortable with technology than others, but all nurses must advocate a balance between "working with technology and providing hands-on nursing" (Casetta, 1993b). Nurses must certainly remain in touch with the cutting edge of technology, but not to the extent of replacing the human responses of caring (Peck, 1992). In many situations, nurses have felt that advanced technology may distance them from patients because they need to pay such extensive attention to the equipment. However, with data derived from such equipment, critical information can be retrieved that allows nurses to focus on caring while also "being with" the patient.

Fenton (1986) described the practice of nursing as two dichotomous and distinct functions: (a) expressive/supportive competence and (b) technological competence. This perceived dichotomy isolates technology from caring, thereby preempting any realization of their coexistence and interdependence. Such technological competence is expressed as technical achievement in practice. Being supportive and expressive is one of the ways in which caring is demonstrated and enhances the humanness of technological proficiency. I believe that being technologically masterful can be considered the expressive/supportive exhibition of nursing as demonstrated through caring. When the nurse uses technology as an aid to knowing the patient as a caring person, rather than focusing on the technology per se, the process of nursing is enhanced.

This chapter presents, as interdependent entities, technology, caring, and extant theoretical perspectives of caring and technology in nursing. Three perspectives will be explained: (a) technological caring (Ray, 1987), (b) technology dependency (Sandelowski, 1993), and (c) technology and caring coexisting in nursing (Locsin, 1994). From these caring and technology perspectives, the model of caring technology will be described, illuminating the power of technology and caring in nursing.

TECHNOLOGY

In relation to the practice of nursing, technology, the first of these three key concepts, is viewed as a means to an end and as a human activity (Heidegger, 1977). Fenton (1986) declared that nursing has been traditionally described as either task-oriented (the dependence that competent nurse actions have on instrumental and technical functioning) or care-oriented (the expressive, supportive, or person-oriented functions that are often required during illness and hospitalization). As means to an end, activities like procuring and utilizing exist as processes while simultaneously responding to a human activity. Within this framework is instrumentality: the fundamental characteristic of technology that is explained as "every attempt to bring human beings into right relation to technology. Everything depends on our manipulating technology in the proper manner as means" (Heidegger, 1977, p. 17).

Technology in nursing is also broadly perceived to include computer literacy and robotic proficiency. Technology allows nurses to know and assist the patient more fully toward well-being (Peck, 1992). On the other hand, computers and other health care technologies have the potential to interfere with nurses' decisions and abilities to confirm patients as persons. These technologies can divert nurses away from providing the quality of care that is personally confirming to patients (Menix, 1993). As exemplified in the process of rehabilitation, Platts and Fraser (1993) likened technology to the skillful manipulation of assisting functions for patients, particularly in relation to mobility (e.g., wheelchairs and cars), functionality (e.g., page turning or the possession of robotic arms), communication (e.g., keyboard emulators or voice processors), and control of the environment. Hudson (1993) alludes to technology as "curing," with an emphasis on technological and physical competence. Reilly and Behrens-Hanna (1991) refer to technology as that aspect of care which addresses moral and ethical issues inherent in the practice of nursing. This issue may refer to nursing actions that sustain biological functions without regard for living as the patient envisions it.

Some clinical situations exemplify the valuing of technology in clinical evaluations and decisions. One of these situations is described by Pierson and Funk (1989), who found that data made available by a pulmonary artery catheter were in no instance identified as factors used to determine fluid management decisions; rather, data obtained by noninvasive clinical evaluations like urine output, chest X-ray, and edema were used as bases. Such results raise questions regarding the legitimacy of various patient "technologies." The impact of technology in nursing practice is well demonstrated by Cooper's (1993) consecration of the intensive care unit (ICU) as the ultimate place where technology is experienced. She said that "nowhere is the nature of technology more evident than in the microculture of an intensive care unit (ICU), where the dominance of technology renders many experiences invisible. ICUs are inescapably distinguished and defined by technology" (p. 24). As the ultimate environment for technologically proficient nurses, the ICU justifies delineations between empathy as caring and technology as curing (Hudson, 1993). Various descriptions of technology allude to its "reign" in nursing, which characterizes it as never disappearing.

The intensive care unit as the definitive locale of technology is supported by an experienced nurse who exclaimed that "oftentimes what people see are ICU nurses who are focusing a lot on the machines because machines are giving tremendous bodily physical support to that patient. The machines are actually fundamental for us in this kind of unit" (Cooper, 1993, p. 26). Further evidence of this perception of the ICU was noted as early as the 1950s: "The nurses did not consider familiar equipment and machines 'technology.' To them, technology represented 'new' science, machines (such as dialysis machines and heart monitors) that were complex and actually sustained patients or provided previously unobtainable data" (Fairman, 1992, p. 57). The power of technology as a means to an end and as a human activity was set, not because of equipment or the availability of instruments, but because of the intensity of the technology that was needed to sustain and/or maintain human life. Competence in triage

(sorting and grouping patients) and the complexity of the observation that transpires 24 hours a day through the vigilance of nurses demonstrate this intensity
in emergency and trauma situations as well as in critical care areas.

Technique and *technology* are familiar terms that tend to be perceived as dilut-
ing the impact of nursing activities in health care. As conciliatory concepts, these
are explained with the underpinnings of utilization in nursing practice. Zwolski
(1989) describes technique as "simply a standard method that can be taught, a
recipe that can be duplicated, and if followed, will always lead to the desired end,
whereas technology is the embodiment of technique" (p. 238). As such, it can be
recognized by its methods and expressions, such as in reproductive technology.
Techniques like fetal monitoring, in vitro fertilization, and artificial insemina-
tion are easily identified as aspects of reproduction technology (Zwolski, 1989).

Technology in nursing, according to Jacox, Pillar, and Redman (1990), is
important if nursing is to be understood as a human activity and as a means to
promote the well-being of patients. From definitions of nursing to definitions
of allied health professions, Jacox et al. (1990) have argued the need to classify
those technologies that nursing practitioners use. Although the issue of ownership of a particular technology consistently instigates academic discussions between and among proponent owners, these authors succinctly stress that "if a
technology is used by more than one discipline, that technology is not owned by
any single profession, nor can any single profession claim the sole right to be re-
imbursed for the technology" (p. 84). Therefore, the question for nursing is the
following: What technologies comprise unique nursing technologies? Although
they list a taxonomy of nursing technologies, Jacox et al. (1990) nonetheless
acknowledge that this list is "not intended to encompass all of nurses' activities,
but only to list examples of [the] technologies" (p. 82). Their list offers useful
examples of technologies as means to an end and as human activity. These technologies bring the nurse into a relational encounter with the patient to facilitate the living of each other's hopes, dreams, and aspirations as person. In
summary, the purpose of technology in nursing is not just to retrieve data,
achieve particular status among health care providers, or simply exhibit proficiency, but rather, and most importantly, to intentionally know the person as
living and growing in caring.

CARING CONCEPTS IN NURSING PRACTICE

Let us focus now on the impact of the second concept, caring in nursing practice. The regard for caring as nursing's "special knowledge" has been claimed by
Olson (1993) as the path that professionalization of nursing must follow in
order to establish itself as a full-fledged profession. Porter (1992) supports this

by emphasizing that "one of the most consistent strategies to achieve professionalization for nursing has been the attempt to acquire a unique knowledge
base" (p. 72). The possession of such knowledge is seen as one of the essential
traits of a "true" profession. The influence of caring in nursing is reaching a
level of sophistication that supports the realization of nursing as a discipline
and profession.

Issues that emerge about caring in nursing include caring as the essence of
nursing, caring as the tradition of nursing, and caring as a process of interaction and communication in nursing. As the essence of nursing, Leininger
(1984) explains caring as "the central, dominant and unifying feature of nursing" (p. 152). Lynaugh and Fagin (1988) claim that caring is the common link
that brings nurses together. Watson (1985) stresses that caring is the moral
ideal of nursing, and Roach (1987) considers caring as "the human mode of
being" (p. ix). These descriptions forge the important position of caring as not
unique to nursing but rather as unique *in* nursing.

To address the issue that caring has traditionally constituted nursing practice activities, Olson (1993) studied achievement evaluations of nurses at St.
Luke's Hospital (London, England) from 1915 to 1937. She found that the performance of nurses was frequently evaluated and rated in terms of how they
"controlled," "managed," and "handled" patients toward a discernible outcome
of "neat, finished-appearing work" (p. 71). These activities were more valuable
to nursing supervisors than those that reflected person-oriented actions. But
putting more weight on skills and outcomes in the overall evaluations of nursing care, rather than on evidence for showing concern toward patients as persons, contradicts the traditional claim that nursing practice constitutes caring.

On the issue of interaction and communication, Noddings (1984) explained
that caring occurs when one is completely receptive to another. This depiction
is shared by Phillips (1993), who described caring as an interactive process that
requires the carer to be responsive to the needs of the person cared for. The interactive nature of caring as simply "coresponsiveness" is a simplistic way of
showing nursing as it transpires between the nurse and the person being nursed.

The meaning of caring in nursing practice is expanded to include two integral
concepts: (a) duty to care for others and (b) the right of the nurse to control her
or his own activities in the name of caring. As Reverby (1987) succinctly expressed, nurses are expected to act out of an obligation or duty to care, taking on
caring more as an identity than as work, and expressing humanitarianism without thought of autonomy either at the bedside or in their profession. The concepts
of the duty to care and the right to own one's activities have influenced many
contemporary issues of political empowerment strategies that affect organizational
change, particularly in nursing. Situations in which nursing occurs have been
described as the "caring moment" (Watson, 1985), the "now moment" (Parse,

1987), the "between" (Paterson & Zderad, 1988), and the "caring between" (Boykin & Schoenhofer, 1993).

Nursing's educational philosophy, ideological underpinnings, and structured positions have made it difficult to create circumstances within which to gain recognition for caring values. Nurses continue to struggle with issues regarding the basis for and the value of caring. The articulation of nursing as a practice discipline has become the dominant cry in the further development of nursing. Theories of nursing grounded in caring offer a perspective from which to view the discipline.

THEORETICAL PERSPECTIVES OF CARING TECHNOLOGY

In this section, three theoretical perspectives that structure the study of caring technology in nursing are discussed: (a) technological caring (Ray, 1987), technology dependency (Sandelowski, 1993), and coexistence of technology and caring in nursing (Locsin, 1995).

The concept of technological caring was coined by Ray (1987). As a result of her work in critical care, she describes the ethical process of believing in the power of technology to change or reverse the patient's state or to influence nurses' decisions to allow a patient to live or die peacefully, coupled with moral reasoning that focuses on obligations to "do no harm (beneficence and non-maleficence), to be fair (justice), and to allow choice (autonomy)" (p. 170). Because critical care nurses usually work to sustain life, these experiential ethical shifts are important for a fuller understanding of the meaning of caring. In order to make the shifts, three operative processes were described: "1) the dominant values of the critical care nurse who believed in technology and treatment; 2) how the uses of technology were interpreted; and 3) the extent of patient suffering" (p. 170). These processes operate on the ethico-moral aspects of reasoning in technological caring, but compassion is what motivates the change "in the ethical decision-making process of technological caring" (Ray, 1994, personal communication, College of Nursing, Florida Atlantic University, April 13, 1994). This is the unity of meaning between the experience of critical care and technological caring, which has its foundation in ethics, the coexistent relationship between experience and principle (Ray, 1987). Figure 3–1 shows Ray's (1987) model of the meaning of critical care nursing.

Utilizing Bush's (1983) definition of technology as "people, tools, and techniques in organized systems of interaction to achieve human goals" (p. 36), Sandelowski (1993) introduced the theory of technology dependency: "that

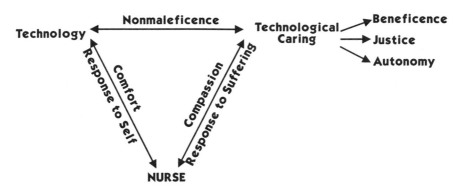

Figure 3–1   Model of the meaning of critical care nursing: Technological caring as experiential and principle-based ethics (Ray, 1987, p. 170). Copyright © 1986, Marilyn A. Ray.

short- or long-term reliance on devices and techniques to evaluate or satisfy or resolve health-related needs or problems" (p. 37). "People" are described as those involved in the invention, dissemination, application, and use of technology. These individuals include the recipients of health care services, nurses, physicians, technicians, sales representatives, and repair personnel. "Tools," in Bush's definition, include devices, instruments, and machines, from thermometers to computerized tomography (CT) scanners; "technique" refers to the procedures that put tools to clinical use, such as venipuncture, cardiac catheterization, and surgery. Sandelowski described the existence of a view that perceives humanity's dependence on technology. This existence has intended and unintended outcomes based on operations and intervening processes. Although technology dependency is appreciated as existing in order to know the patients through the recognition and proposition of possible independence from technology, reliance on nontechnological means to evaluate and/or satisfy/resolve health needs/problems can be acknowledged. Figure 3–2, a concept map of technology dependency in health care, delineates the processes of technology dependency and independency (Sandelowski, 1993).

The perspective of technology and caring as coexisting in nursing is grounded in the model "nursing as caring." This perspective describes the focus of nursing as "nurturing persons living caring and growing in caring" (Boykin & Schoenhofer, 1993, p. 21). From the perspective of nursing as caring, all nursing takes place in nursing situations, that is, "shared lived experiences in which the caring between nurse and nursed enhances personhood" (p. 24). Within the intimacy of the nursing situation, calls for nursing are first expressed, heard, and addressed. Calls are conceptualized in the mind of the nurse as she or he enters the world of the other with the intention of knowing the

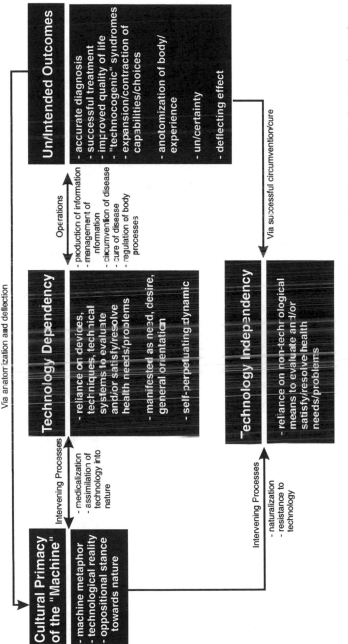

Cultural Primacy of the "Machine"

- machine metaphor
- technological reality
- oppositional stance towards nature

Intervening Processes
- medicalization
- assimilation of technology into nature

Technology Dependency

- reliance on devices, techniques, technical systems to evaluate and/or satisfy/resolve health needs/problems

- manifested as need, desire, general orientation

- self-perpetuating dynamic

Operations
- production of information
- management of information
- circumvention of disease
- cure of disease
- regulation of body processes

Un/Intended Outcomes

- accurate diagnosis
- successful treatment
- improved quality of life
- "technocogenic" syndromes
- expansion/contraction of capabilities/choices

- anotomization of body/ experience

- un/certainty

- deflecting effect

Via anatomization and deflection

Via successful circumvention/cure

Technology Independency

- reliance on non-technological means to evaluate an d/or satisfy/resolve health needs/problems

Intervening Processes
- naturalization
- resistance to technology

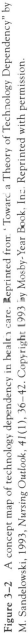

Figure 3-2   A concept map of technology dependency in health care. Reprinted from 'Toward a Theory of Technology Dependency" by M. Sandelowski, 1993, *Nursing Outlook, 41*(1), 36–42. Copyright 1993 by Mosby-Year Book, Inc. Reprinted with permission.

other as caring person. These calls arise from an understanding of the person's unique ways of living caring in the moment and of expressing dreams and aspirations for growing as caring person. Calls for nursing are calls to be known and affirmed as caring person. Nursing responses are specific forms of caring that are created within the uniqueness of the situation. Personhood, the process of living grounded in caring, is enhanced in the shared experience of the nursing situation. Nursing is "the intentional and authentic presence of the nurse with another who is known as person living caring and growing in caring" (p. 25). With caring as process, the person grows in competence to express the self as caring. Because technology is part of the wholeness of the person, and with caring as process, nursing can be conceived as the nurse's caring process demonstrated as proficiency in technology while being with the person.

In order to appreciate technological competence in caring, its utilization as a means to an end and as a human activity (Heidegger, 1977) must be personified with evidence and proofs of intentionality and technological responsibility, while supported with a theoretical model of nursing. The professional nurse is challenged to be technologically masterful and still respond authentically and intentionally to calls for nursing. Authenticity and intentionality are demonstrated when the nurse accepts the patient (with all the demands of technological expertise) and attempts to know the patient fully as person in the process of living his or her hopes, dreams, and aspirations. Burfitt, Greiner, Miers, Kinney, and Branyon (1993) describe caring for critically ill patients as a "mutual process in which intentions are joined to form a shared experience. In this mutual process, healing is an outcome that might otherwise be elusive" (p. 489). In the context of nursing as caring, healing is understood in the sense of recognizing, rather than restoring, wholeness (Schoenhofer, 1994, personal communication, College of Nursing, Florida Atlantic University, July 31, 1994).

Figure 3–3 explains the relationships among the concepts of technology, caring, and competence, while "nursing as caring" provides the theoretical perspective of technology and caring coexisting in nursing. Considered as independent entities, technology and caring may thus coexist in discord. This is typically exemplified by the role of nonprofessional nurses, regarded by Phillips (1993) as nurses of the lower orders in nursing, who are being renamed care assistants, indicating differences of status between nursing and caring. This description of types of caregivers perpetuates the effects of language that tends to dichotomize caring and technology, thus fostering the existence of their paradoxical relationship. A nurse who performs technology proficiently without knowing the patient as a person is the ultimate portrait of one who is simply *doing* technology. This visionary expression illuminates the power of technology and caring in nursing.

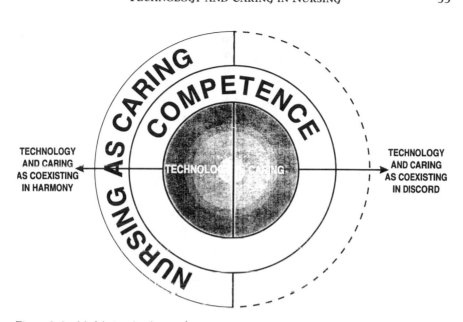

Figure 3-3 Model of technology and caring in nursing. Copyright © 1993, Rozzano C. Locsin.

STRUCTURING THE POWER OF CARING TECHNOLOGY IN NURSING

Caring technology is the unifying, compelling attraction that exists between technology and caring in nursing. This is illustrated in Figure 3–4 as a continuous line that traverses the circular unity of the structure, emerging and represented as a "yin and yang" configuration that characterizes the continuing reliance of contemporary health care on technology and caring. This image exemplifies current nursing practice as dependent on technology while espousing the necessity to express concern for persons as human beings, by retaining the perception of patients not as objects but as persons (Gadow, 1984). Although it depends on the impact of technology to know the person as person, the caring perspective of humanness enhances this codependency rather than simply depending on technology or on caring alone. The powerful coexistence of these concepts alludes to the relational authenticity of various perspectives, as delineated by the three circles (representing the extant theoretical perspectives) that determine the interconnectedness of technology and caring (see Figure 3–4). The demarcation line between technology and caring in each of these symbols refers to the extent of emphasis between technology and caring. Technological

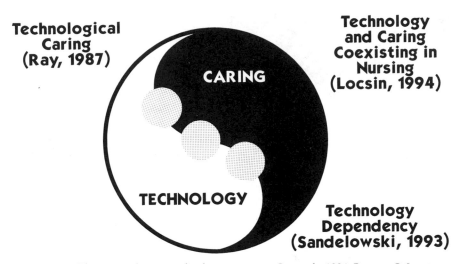

Technological Caring (Ray, 1987)

Technology and Caring Coexisting in Nursing (Locsin, 1994)

CARING

TECHNOLOGY

Technology Dependency (Sandelowski, 1993)

Figure 3–4   The power of caring technology in nursing. Copyright 1994, Rozzano C. Locsin.

caring focuses on the ethico-moral conditions of caring in critical areas; technological dependency focuses on the potency of the force that extends between valuing technology and caring. The perception that technology and caring are coexisting in nursing attempts to instigate conceptualizations about technology as an expression of caring in nursing.

Although these theoretical perspectives demonstrate relationships between technology and caring and refer to their coexistence in nursing, the conceptualization of caring technology is the driving force behind knowing the client intentionally and authentically as person, and it continues to generate explanations for the practice of nursing. An emerging issue in the study of technology and caring in nursing is the consideration of technology as nursing expression (as a means to an end and as human activity), with caring as the "object" of nursing. This exemplifies "technology of nursing" with caring as the ultimate circumstance.

Although this issue has not reached a level of sophistication that demands concurrent clarification, the issue of "nursing as technology" has reached a level of recognition that deserves further explication, if nursing is to insist that it exists as a viable, vital, and integral element in the attainment or maintenance of quality health and care. As Cooper (1993) argued, "Technology is designed to be invincible, invulnerable, objective, and predictable, in contrast to the human characteristics of vulnerability, subjectivity, and unpredictability. It is in this context that the nurse is challenged to care" (p. 26). Herein lies the paradoxical exhibition of technology and caring in nursing. Such caring technology has the power to facilitate the view of persons as human beings rather than as objects. People possess values of dignity and autonomy, and strive to live their hopes, dreams, and aspirations as caring persons. The model of caring technology interprets the living of caring while practicing nursing. Caring is, after all, critical to the contemporary understanding of the value of technology in nursing practice.

REFERENCES

Boykin, A., & Schoenhofer, S. (1993). *Nursing as caring: A model for transforming practice*. New York: National League for Nursing Press.

Burfitt, S., Greiner, D., Miers, L., Kinney, M., & Branyon, M. (1993). Professional nurse caring as perceived by critically ill patients: A phenomenologic study. *American Journal of Critical Care, 2*(6), 489–499.

Bush, C. G. (1983). Women and the assessment of technology: To think, to be, to unthink, to free. In J. Rothschilds (Ed.), Machina ex dea: Feminist perspectives on technology. In Sandelowski, M. (1993). Toward a theory of technology dependency. *Nursing Outlook, 41*(1), 36–42.

Casetta, R. (1993a, November–December). The evolution of high-tech nursing. *The American Nurse*, 18–19.

Casetta, R. (1993b, November–December). Nurses advocate for ethical decisions in high-tech care. *The American Nurse*, 30.

Cooper, M. (1993). The intersection of technology and care in the ICU. *Advances in Nursing Science, 15*(3), 23–32.

Fairman, J. (1992). Watchful vigilance: Nursing care, technology, and the development of intensive care units. *Nursing Research, 41*(1), 56–60.

Fenton, M. (1986). Development of the scale of humanistic nursing behavior. *Nursing Research, 36*(2), 82–87.

Gadow, S. (1984). Touch and technology: Two paradigms of patient care. *Journal of Religion and Health, 23*, 63–69.

Heidegger, M. (1977). *The question concerning technology and other essays*. New York: Harper & Row.

Hudson, G. (1993). Empathy and technology in the coronary care unit. *Intensive Critical Care Nursing, 9*(1), 55–61.

Jacox, A., Pillar, B., & Redman, B. (1990). A classification of nursing technology. *Nursing Outlook, 38*(2), 81–85.

Leininger, M. (Ed.). (1984). *Care: The essence of nursing and health*. Thorofare, NJ: Slack.

Locsin, R. (1995). Machine technologies and caring in nursing. *Image: The Journal of Nursing Scholarship.*

Lynaugh, J., & Fagin, C. (1988). Nursing outcomes of age. *Image: The Journal of Nursing Scholarship, 20,* 184.

Menix, K. (1993). Technology: Complementing or controlling care? *The International Nurse News and Views, 7*(1), 1–6.

Noddings, N. (1984). *Caring: A feminine approach to ethics and moral education.* Berkeley: University of California Press.

Olson, T. (1993). Laying claim to caring: Nursing and the language of training, 1915–1937. *Nursing Outlook, 41*(2), 68–72.

Paterson, J., & Zderad, P. (1988). *Humanistic nursing.* New York: National League for Nursing Press.

Parse, R. (1987). *Nursing science: Major paradigms, theories, and critiques.* Philadelphia: Saunders.

Peck, M. (1992). The future of nursing in a technological age: Computers, robots, and TLC. *Journal of Holistic Nursing, 10*(2), 183–191.

Phillips, P. (1993). A deconstruction of caring. *Journal of Advanced Nursing, 18,* 1554–1558.

Pierson, M., & Funk, M. (1989). Technology versus clinical evaluation for fluid management decisions in CABG patients. *Image: The Journal of Nursing Scholarship, 21*(4), 192–195.

Platts, R., & Fraser, M. (1993). Assistive technology in the rehabilitation of patients with high spinal cord lesions. *Paraplegia, 31*(5), 280–287.

Porter, S. (1992). The poverty of professionalization: A critical analysis of strategies for the occupational advancement of nursing. *Journal of Advanced Nursing, 17,* 723–728.

Ray, M. (1987). Technological caring: A new model in critical care. *Dimensions of Critical Care Nursing, 6*(3), 169–173.

Reilly, D., & Behrens-Hanna, L. (1991). Perioperative nursing: Moral and ethical issues in high-technology practice. *Today's OR Nurse, 13*(8), 10–15.

Reverby, S. (1987). A caring dilemma: Womanhood and nursing in historical perspective. *Nursing Research, 36*(1), 5–11.

Roach, S. (1987). *The human act of caring.* Ottawa: Canadian Hospital Association.

Sandelowski, M. (1993). Toward a theory of technology dependency. *Nursing Outlook, 41*(1), 36–42.

Watson, J. (1985). *Nursing: The philosophy and science of caring.* Boulder, CO: Colorado Associated University Press.

Zwolski, K. (1989). Professional nursing in a technical system. *Image: The Journal of Nursing Scholarship, 21*(4), 238–242.

4

Windows of Opportunity: Caring in Changing Political Climates

Carol Picard
Galina Perfiljeva

> Windows for gazing,
> raising, for air, light and view,
> for dreaming
> windows in our homes and in our hearts
> a gathering of fire stoked
> and watched through the pane of the wood burning stove
> windows on the world
> take what is seen and improve it
> add vision to change the landscape and the future
> join hands to this work with broad brush strokes early
> a palette mixing color, using all the tubes but carefully
> a window portrait of hope.

Opportunities to come together with international colleagues change over time. In one period, some windows may open while others close, only to have the order mix, reconfigure, and change once more. The bodies politic is a living, breathing organism, and its climates and realities influence our professional and personal relationships. We are living in a period of momentous change, as witnessed recently by the South African election and by changes in eastern Europe over the past five years. The proverb "Opportunity is not a lengthy visitor" instructs us to be ready to act, to hear the call for the need to care. It is time to look out the open window.

Dr. Madeline Leininger (1993), who has mentored and supported international nurses for over three decades, is a role model for nurses to collaborate internationally. She has challenged us to create global caring communities with our nurse colleagues. Ten years ago, this chapter would probably not have been possible. To present it together, as coauthors, is a dream fulfilled. Changes in Russia have created opportunities for the advancement of nursing, as well as dangers because of diminishing resources as the country's economy moves to a free market system. The chance for freer access and travel for its citizens has enabled a dialogue between Russian and non-Russian nurses with greater frequency than prior to 1989. What this opportunity presents is a challenge—a challenge to respond to the call for care. This chapter addresses the concerns and needs of nurses in the Russian Federation and ways in which Western nurses can respond to a call for care.

THE RUSSIAN FEDERATION

The Russian Federation is the largest country in the world. It stretches from the Baltic Sea in the West to the Pacific Ocean in the East. The total area of the country is 17 million square kilometers. In 1993, the population totaled 143 million, 74% of whom live in urban areas. The country is undergoing a period of great political, social, and economic changes that influence all areas of society. The health care system is not immune to these changes, and many problems that were denied by the old regime have been revealed. Poor standards and low-quality care, lack of resources, high morbidity and mortality rates, consumer dissatisfaction, and lack of choice are just a few of these problems (World Health Organization, 1992). The Russian Federation faces the challenge of improving health care. Because nurses are the largest group of health care professionals and the quality of nursing is a crucial determinant of the quality of health care as a whole, the need to develop nursing education, practice, and management is of vital importance to meeting the challenges of the changes in society and in health care.

HEALTH STATUS

Numerous social conflicts that have broken out in the country have adversely affected public health. The growing psychological stress on individual citizens and families is reflected in rising divorce rates and falling marriage rates. Life expectancy has declined over the past few years after a rapid increase in 1985–1986. In the first half of 1993, life expectancy was 67.2 years. With a death rate of 12.2 per 1,000 population and a birth rate of 9.1 per 1,000 in the first half of 1993, the population growth of the nation is negative. Infant and maternal mortality rates are high compared to other countries of western Europe. In 1992, the infant mortality rate was 18 deaths per 1,000 live births. The maternal mortality rates remained high—an average of 51 per 100,000 births, with wide regional variation, from 14 in the area of Novgogrod to 107 in Siberia. There are more than 3.5 million abortions per year in the country. In 1992, the ratio of abortions to live births was 225:100, or 98.1 per 1,000 reproductive age women. Abortion is the most common form of family planning (World Health Organization, 1994).

Because of worsening conditions, the rates of most diseases have increased. Many infants are suffering from infectious diseases such as measles and whooping cough. The incidence of salmonella is growing. In 1991, an outbreak of diphtheria reached epidemic proportions (World Health Organization, 1994).

RUSSIAN HEALTH CARE SERVICES

In 1992 and 1993, the functioning of health care services was severely disrupted by inadequate funding and by labor, capital, and supply problems. The Russian Federation health budget was 6.2% of the total state budget—below the budget of 1991 in real terms, and about half the amount required to maintain minimal standards of service provision. Real investment in health systems has dropped by about 50% from its 1991 level. In its attempts to eliminate deficits, the central government is trying to shift budget responsibilities for health onto regional and city governments. In well-endowed localities, this might be possible, but in most cases, lower-level government is unable to make the expected contribution. In 1992, there were 21,000 health care settings in the country, with inpatient care provided by 12,599 hospitals. The average length of stay in the hospital was long: 17 days.

Only 20% of health services are well equipped; 30% are only modestly equipped, and some 50% lack basic equipment and supplies. Hospitals and clinics are forced to function without enough medications, anesthetics, instruments, bandages and linen, X-ray film, and food. Until recently, there was no form of health insurance. Three years ago, the Russian Federation instituted initiatives for health insurance, but little progress has been made to date.

The wages of health personnel have been kept low, which has adversely affected morale and productivity and has generated unprecedented strike actions.

Many health workers have left the health sector and changed professions. Most of them were doctors. The number of doctors has dropped from 46.9 per 10,000 in 1990 to 43.8 per 10,000 in 1992. Because of poor conditions and low standards of life, there are no doctors in 15% of the rural district hospitals. Nurses and *feldshers* (health care workers whose role resembles that of a physician's assistant) now do the doctors' work.

These negative trends in the quality of Russian health care have not been offset by the increase in sophisticated treatment in private facilities, which only a minority can afford.

NURSING IN THE RUSSIAN FEDERATION

The health care system is overstaffed with physicians who are categorized as "higher medical personnel," but many of them perform tasks that in other countries are undertaken by nurses. In 1992, there were 650,000 physicians in the Russian Federation. Nurses comprise half of the middle-level personnel category. The ratio of physicians to nurses is 1:1.5. In some regions, it is even less. There is a widespread shortage of appropriately trained nurses and an oversupply of doctors.

Nearly 95% of the nursing workforce is female. The status and income of nurses are extremely low, hovering just above the poverty line. Most nurses hold down two jobs, to make ends meet.

Nurses do not practice autonomously unless they are working in areas where no physician is available. Their working conditions are poor, and the workload is exceedingly demanding. Nurses have merely followed doctors' orders with few opportunities to make decisions. Nursing is therefore dependent on and subordinate to medicine, and most doctors believe this is right and proper.

By law, nursing duties are listed as follows: caring for patients; care of the body; diet; bedding; assistance in emergencies; observation of weight, pulse, temperature, respiration, skin color, excretion, and psychological condition; carrying out medical instructions regarding medications; intramuscular or subcutaneous injections; lavage; probing; preoperative preparation; monitoring of anesthesia; dressings; assistance in therapeutic and diagnostic activities; collaboration in pre- and posttherapeutic intervention; health education; and maintenance of medico-technical equipment.

There is no licensing of nursing practice except where a license is required for private practice. A new state system of qualification verification was introduced in 1992 for nurses who have more than three years' experience in nursing practice. It consists of an oral examination which, if successful, results in a higher grade and an increase in salary. Three grades of qualification result from passing the relevant examination: second, first, and highest. These qualifications are registered by the Qualifications Commissions nominated by the Ministry.

Nursing education is medically oriented and under medical control. The directors of nursing schools are physicians; nurses and *feldshers* make up only 6% of the teaching staff. Most students enter training at the age of 17, after 11 years of schooling. There is no upper limit for entry into nurses' training. Until recently, there was only one level of nursing education, a two-year basic course with various opportunities for short-term specialization or refresher courses (averaging 1 to 2 months.) Nursing education had no advancement in the past. Nurses could not reach their full potential in contributing to health because they lacked the resources of training materials. They had very few useful textbooks, and materials tended to be medically oriented, with little or no discussion of caring skills, primary health care, or health promotion. Any foreign textbook is still highly prized, regardless of its relevance. Some aid agencies have been sending textbooks to Russia, but their usefulness to students is limited because of language barriers. Often, the content is not suited to their needs. Qualified nurses have no books or journals to keep their knowledge and practice up-to-date. As a result, many nurses were so dissatisfied that they left the profession, many within a few years.

THE NEED FOR CHANGE IN NURSING IN RUSSIA

Nurses in the Russian Federation are the largest group of employees in the national health care system. The quality of nursing is the crucial determinant of the quality of health care as a whole. Because nurses provide direct care to patients, their actions influence both quality of care and patients' perceptions of care. Effectiveness, efficiency, and humanity—the cornerstones of high-quality service—depend to a large extent on the work of nurses. As the national debt continues to rise and places more economic pressures on health care budgets, provision of the most cost-effective and efficient care is vital. Nurses can potentially save hospitals a great deal of money. Adequate care can reduce complications (such as wound infections and pressure sores) and the length of stay in hospitals. A focus on health promotion as part of a nursing model is necessary to expand out of the medical model of nursing education, which has been practiced in the country for many decades. A few years ago, a small group of Russian nursing students went to Germany as part of a health care exchange visit. They were anxious to show the Germans their knowledge of treatments for decubiti and asked the director of nurses to see a patient with this medical problem. The chief nurse left and, when she returned some time later, she told the students she had arranged for a bus to take them to another hospital to see a patient with a decubitus, since this hospital had none. The shocked students came away with an awareness of what prevention can do in nursing situations. Nursing skills can be employed to promote a quick recovery or an early discharge from the hospital. Nurses working daily with patients in the community can prevent illnesses and make it unnecessary for people to go to a hospital in the first place.

The need to improve nursing has been recognized widely in the country. Upgrading of nursing education and preparation of nurse teachers in concepts basic to nursing practice have been identified as of vital importance of health care reform.

Lack of leadership skills has also been recognized as a barrier to managing the changes in the health care system and in the development of nursing. Nurses need to develop management and leadership skills in order to achieve effective and efficient performance, to meet the challenges in the society and in health care, and to become a greater force in directing health care policy in Russia.

Despite difficult circumstances, progress has been made in nursing education. A new curriculum was prepared by the Ministry of Health and circulated to all 340 basic nursing schools. Following the recommendations of the first WHO European Conference on Nursing, held in Vienna in 1988 (World Health Organization, 1989), this curriculum will prepare a nurse of the future for a role that includes not only hospital nursing but also much more responsibility for primary care nursing.

In the period from 1991 to 1993, new advanced 3–4-year programs were introduced in 48 nursing colleges, to prepare graduates who would be able to practice at an advanced level. There are active attempts to introduce the nursing process into the courses, but the lack of qualified teachers and teaching materials is a major obstacle to progress.

There are 40 postbasic nursing schools and 50 departments of basic nursing schools providing short courses of continuing education. More than 100 different postbasic training programs, lasting from 2 weeks to 6 months, enable nurses to practice in specialized nursing fields such as physiotherapy, pediatrics, intensive care, and surgery. Hospitals also put on study days, similar to U.S. continuing education programs.

The first university-based master's course in nursing began at the Moscow Medical Academy in 1991. The four-year, full-time course is aimed at preparing qualified nurses for the future leadership positions in nursing education and management. The students need to develop the competencies of management science and a repertoire of administrative skills in addition to their fundamental knowledge and nursing skills. Since 1991, nine other university-based programs in nursing have been established in Russia. They are linked into a network to share experiences and to learn from each other. A few successful attempts have been made to undertake nursing research. Master's courses lack experienced, appropriately trained faculty and learning materials, but it is a beginning in the plan to advance nursing. Partnerships with experienced Western colleagues, with nursing schools and nursing organizations, are needed like never before. Nurses in Russia face an enormous challenge in trying to strengthen the nursing contribution to health care.

CURRENT PRIORITIES FOR RUSSIAN NURSING

The following are priorities for nursing in the Russian Federation: development of a national action plan for nursing and midwifery; development of nursing leadership; reform of nursing and midwifery education; clinical demonstration projects to create models of good practice; improvement of nurse networking and information systems; development of partnerships with Western colleagues (World Health Organization, 1994).

RESOURCES OF WESTERN NURSES: CREATING CARING WINDOWS

Nurses in the West have access to greater resources than Russian colleagues do: telecommunications, literature, research, supplies of all kinds are at our disposal for education practice and research. As Maya Angelou (1994), the American poet, reminded an audience in Boston, our passage has been paid for. Someone has paid the price for the resources we enjoy today, and our obligation is to give in measure to what we have been given. Creating a global caring community for nurses is one way of doing this. Some might say that our own resources aren't all that great and we could use care ourselves. It is all a matter of perspective. There is a story of a Texan who went to Ireland and met an Irish farmer. The Irishman was proud to show his visitor his modest plot of land. Once finished this brief tour, he asked the Texan, "Do you have a farm?" The Texan boasted, "Well, if I get in my car and I drive all day, if I am lucky, by sundown, I reach the other end of my property." The Irish host paused thoughtfully, looked up at the sky, and mused, "Yes, I had a car like that once." It is all a matter of perspective.

Sister Simone Roach's (1992) attributes of caring are the elements required in creating a global caring relationship. Elements of compassion, competence, commitment, confidence, and conscience are needed to create a global caring community. Karl (1992) described caring as creating a holding environment for our patients. Russian colleagues need Western nurses to find a way to create a holding environment for them, in small and large ways, so that they might create the change they are committed to in nursing. Sister Simone's attributes of caring are elements in this holding environment. Our *compassion* must be informed by a growing awareness of the lived experience of nurses in other countries. For example, federal nurses in Russia who work at what is equivalent to the U.S. National Institutes of Health have not been paid for three months because of budget shortfalls. Basic resources to institute change are unavailable, but nurses still believe they can change this system. We must be *competent* in knowing how to help first, by listening carefully to the call for care, by learning about the resources available, and by linking together and passing the word. The importance of listening to the call for care is so important. Recently, a group of nurse consultants told Russian nurses they needed to change the name nurses are called, from *medsistra* to nurse. This recommendation was made without consultation with the nurses as to the history of the name and its importance to those in the profession. Denying cultural context and history was unacceptable to the Russian nurses. We must have a *commitment* to care. While I was visiting Russia in October, several nurses said to me, "Please don't forget us. Many people come and then leave promising to help, but we don't hear from them again." Global caring requires following through, even when one is met with dead-end leads for help, or when staying in contact is a challenge. We need *confidence*, a belief that we can make a difference. Lech Walesa, in a speech to the U.S. Congress, said that there is a declining world market for words (1989). He meant action was necessary to foster and support change in Eastern bloc countries. These differences are being made by individuals and by organizations of all sizes. We must listen for the opportunity, and work at collaborating with one another in these efforts. Our *conscience*, Roach's fifth attribute, requires we do what is needed, not what is easy. We must actively hope for change for our Russian colleagues. Vaclav Havel, the former president of the Czech Republic, said the following about hope:

> Hope is a state of mind, not of the world. . . . Hope, in this deep and powerful sense, is not the same as joy that things are going well, as willingness to invest in enterprises that are obviously headed for success, but rather an ability to work for something because it is good, not just because it stands a chance to succeed. (Symynkyjwicz, 1991, p. 22)

WINDOWS FOR OPPORTUNITIES

Circumstances and people create opportunities. It was my good fortune to serve the Massachusetts Nurses Association when Dr. Perfiljeva came to visit the United States in 1990. Then-president Barbara Stanley asked me to escort a Russian visitor. I had no idea where this service would take me. We come to crossroads where the call to care invites us. Although we did not know then how great the changes would be in her country, we knew the time was right for building a global caring community with Russian nurses.

Max Depree (1991), in his book *Leadership Jazz*, identifies the water carrier as a special kind of leader in an organization, the one who keeps things running, not an identified leader. I am a water carrier. I carry supplies and look for ways to foster growth, sustain change, and link resources for Galina. When Maya Angelou spoke in Boston (1994), she talked about the people in her life who were most important and who had cared for her. When she was about to do something fearful or particularly challenging, she would invite them to join her, if only in spirit, in her heart. I often feel like Galina is in my heart or by my side as I attend conferences or meetings because I am always looking out for resources or possibilities she might find helpful. Depree also believes that to lead is to serve. I think Mr. Depree and Sister Simone are kindred spirits in their orientation to a caring environment.

Dr. Perfiljeva is a visionary. She lives Sr. Simone's attributes of caring in her daily life as a leader of nursing in Russia, and illuminates the path for those nurses struggling for autonomy and a caring environment in which they can practice their profession.

STRATEGIES FOR GLOBAL NURSE CARING

Our goal is to support the advancement of nursing in Russia through education and through professional organizations such as the Moscow City Nurses Association. We can demonstrate care through dialogue on the Internet, support for a nursing journal, sending leaders and scholars to lecture to nursing groups, encouraging student exchanges, sharing materials, and applying to private foundations and the government for funding for joint projects. This isn't easily done. Federal agencies often do not see the wisdom and necessity of advancing nursing education. Agencies are not sure how to respond to such innovations in health care as Dr. Perfiljeva's master's program in nursing. They are puzzled because it does not meet requirements for direct health-related aid and it is not the kind of education-related project they usually target. We must educate our elected officials on how such a project benefits the country as a whole. Perhaps national nursing organizations in our countries need to mobilize nurses to educate our legislators.

Pick your window. The World Health Organization is sponsoring the LEMON project, which needs funds to translate nursing materials into the languages of the countries of Eastern Europe and the Russian Federation. Fitchburg State College has instituted a Center for Mentorship to support joint projects with Russian nurses through telecommunications, student and faculty exchanges, and text translation projects with the Moscow Medical Academy. Many other schools in the Russian Federation are in need of such partnerships with Western colleagues willing to support and promote caring in this time of political change.

CONCLUSION

Nursing knows no boundaries. Nursing is international. In spite of language problems and differing backgrounds, we can still understand and support each other. The future lies in those places where efforts are joined to create possibilities for caring windows to be opened. We can all help to color the landscape beyond the windows of opportunity for global caring in nursing.

REFERENCES

Angelou, M. (1994, April 25). Speech at the Emerson Majestic Theater, Boston, MA.

Depree, M. (1992). *Leadership jazz*. New York: Doubleday.

Karl, Rev. J. C. (1992). Being there: Who do you bring to practice? In D. Gaut (Ed.), *The presence of caring in nursing* (pp. 1–13). New York: National League for Nursing Press.

Leininger, M. (1993). Culture care theory: The comparative global theory to advance human care nursing knowledge and practice. In D. Gaut (Ed.), *A global agenda for caring* (pp. 3–18). New York: National League for Nursing Press.

Roach, S. (1992). *The human act of caring*. Ottawa, Canada: Canadian Hospital Association.

Symynkyjwicz, B. (1991). Vaclav Havel and the politics of hope. *Noetic Sciences Review*, 18–24.

Walesa, L. (1989). Solidarity and freedom. Speech delivered before joint session of Congress. *Vital Speeches of the Day,* November 15, 1989.

World Health Organization. (1989). European conference on nursing: A report of a WHO meeting, Vienna, 21–24 June 1988. Copenhagen: WHO Regional Office for Europe.

World Health Organization. (1992). *Highlights on health in the Russian Federation.* Copenhagen: WHO Regional Office for Europe.

World Health Organization. (1994). *Russian Federation nursing and midwifery profile.* Copenhagen: WHO Regional Office for Europe. Unedited draft.

5

The Power of Caring: Issues and Strategies

Madeleine Leininger

As nurses increase their understanding of diverse cultures and assume leadership roles in a dynamic and changing political, economic, and cultural world, they will come to value the importance of humanistic and scientific caring as the central and essential focus of nursing. Although caring, as the essence of nursing, has not been fully recognized by all nurses, a growing and enthusiastic cadre of care clinicians and scholars are moving forward to establish care as the central, distinct, and unifying domain of knowledge and practice of the nursing discipline. Nurses who value, know, and practice caring realize how meaningful and essential a caring mode of functioning is in assisting people in a variety of human conditions.

A caring ethos and concomitant caring skills have also become essential for understanding and working with people transculturally in diverse environmental contexts. Most importantly, nurses are realizing the need for humanistic care philosophies, theories, and knowledge, if they are to be effective and successful survivors in a competitive and changing economic, political, and cultural world. Transcultural caring knowledge and skills are becoming a powerful force in what I call *The New Age Movement* in nursing education and practice. This new movement supports an open discovery approach and diverse ways of learning and of helping people who have different cultural lifeways and needs.

Discovering and using transcultural caring knowledge and skills is part of the New Age Movement to participate in a global community (Leininger, 1991, 1992, 1995). During the past two decades, a cadre of committed nurse care scholars and nursing associations such as the Transcultural Nursing Society (since 1970), the International Association of Human Caring (since 1978), and, more recently, the National League for Nursing have been moving forward to transform nursing by making care the major focus of nursing and health care (Gaut, 1993; Leininger, 1992, 1995; Watson, 1985).

Transforming nursing education and service systems into a caring philosophy and a mode of functioning has necessitated knowledge and understanding about the realities of different political nursing and cultural contexts. Indeed, this is one of the most critical and challenging issues facing nursing today. Moreover, it is one of the most difficult challenges, largely because of latent professional interests, knowledge, and skills dealing with power phenomena and the politics of caring. In every culture, power and politics play a joint role in shaping, governing, and determining many aspects of human existence, health, wellness, and chronic illnesses. Power and politics can greatly influence illness and caring patterns of cultures in overt and subtle ways. Hence, nurses need to understand the sources and forms of power and politics if they are to succeed in transforming nursing into a quality-based caring profession. Nurses need to become far more knowledgeable about the nature and uses of power if they are to make appropriate decisions and actions bearing on caring in different environmental contexts. Most importantly, the relationship of politics to social-structure factors such as economics, social and kinship ties, legal and religious education, technology, and the specific cultural values and norms of any culture is an essential domain of knowledge if nurses are to function effectively in our multicultural world. Culturally constituted power and politics can literally "make or break" the way nurses function and how they make care a visible and viable way to help consumers. It is safe to say that practically every aspect of caring in nursing has political aspects in the initiation and maintenance of care practices in education and nursing services.

This chapter is focused on identifying some contemporary power and political issues related to dimensions of human caring from a nursing perspective. The purpose is to raise awareness of the covert dimensions of power and politics, in order to help nurses discover and use this knowledge in nursing practice and education. Much is yet to be discovered about power, politics, and caring in different nursing contexts and cultures, especially from a transcultural nursing perspective. As nurses begin to study the power and politics of care, these components are usually embedded in the worldview and in the diverse social structure and organizational dimensions of education and practice. Most nurses have yet to become fully aware of the political culture of nursing, hospitals, and health organizations, and how much that culture influences nursing care practices. The current trends in the United States—downsizing, restructuring, reconfiguring, and making similar changes in hospitals and health organizations—are laden with power and political operational modes. Diverse political maneuvers and strategies have been used to lay off, relocate, reassign, or fire nurses in many settings under the guise of economic and restructuring processes. The cultural shock of these realities has stimulated some nurses to reassess and learn about power and politics in their current and future employment settings.

IDENTIFYING FEATURES OF POWER, POLITICS, AND CARING

At the outset, it is well to clarify the terms being used, in order to promote common understandings of the concepts under discussion. *Power*, in the simplest use, refers to *the ability to influence individuals or groups in their decisions and actions in order to achieve certain goals or purposes* (Kottak, 1991, p. 221). *Politics* refers to *the ability to use available human and material resources in order to regulate and/or manage the affairs and decisions of others*. *Politics* has been defined by Williams (1990) as "the cultural and social patterns humans employ in applying power to make public policy decisions" (p. 410). *Caring* refers to those *assistive, supportive, and facilitative acts for or toward individuals and groups to help them maintain or retain their health (or well being), or to deal with disabilities and handicaps in diverse environmental human conditions* (Leininger, 1988b, 1991).

In every culture, power and politics tend to vary in organizational structures and in the ways these dimensions are expressed with their diverse meanings. Power expressions and politics are closely related to persons in authority or to those who hold influential positions, statuses, or role responsibilities. Moreover, the phenomenon of hegemony may be associated with persons in authority roles who have ascribed or achieved power. *Hegemony* refers to *persons or groups who exert undue or considerable force on others in social or political organizations with the intent to take over or subdue the power of others*. Hegemonic practices can be seen when the rights, responsibilities, and positions of others are taken over suddenly in a very short span of time in order to gain the political authority that exists in the competition for scarce resources, money, and power (Kottak, 1991). Hegemonic practices exist in patriarchal dominated hospitals and health agencies, and in societies searching for control and power over people and physical resources. Hegemonic actions can destroy a system, program, or agency in a very short span of time. The political interests and reasons for hegemonic actions may be baffling to those affected, but are usually planned and well known to the hegemonic political leaders who want something very badly.

In any social or cultural organization, the nurse needs to be knowledgeable about such hegemonic practices and about the multiple social structure factors that can influence establishing and maintaining a caring philosophy and normative caring practices. Power and politics can be found in the social-structure factors related to economics, political and legal education, and technological and cultural value systems in any organization, culture, or society. The difficulty is that power in social-structure factors is usually covert and deeply embedded in different dimensions of the social structure so that it is not readily identifiable. One has to study, observe, and analyze social-structure factors to discover their power and political influences on caring, and to learn how these forces can be used to transform institutions and programs into constructive caring ethos.

Unfortunately, only in recent years have nurses begun serious study of power, politics, and the political dimensions of nursing, even though a few nurse leaders began to be concerned scholars of these areas nearly two decades ago (Ashley, 1977; Kalisch & Kalisch, 1982; Leininger, 1974, 1978; Ray, 1989). Nursing, especially, needs to give far more attention to political structure factors, worldview, and the ethnohistorical context in which nurses function, in order to fully understand the dynamics of power and politics in relation to human caring. Such knowledge is crucial if nursing practices are to have a caring emphasis (Boykin & Schoenhofen, 1993). The current emphasis on empowerment of nurses is helpful, but an in-depth perspective is needed to understand empowerment and its relationship to power sources and political operations. Theoretical perspectives are also needed to study the politics of caring. For example, the theory of Culture Care Diversity and Universality (Leininger, 1991, 1992, 1995) can be most valuable to explicate social structure and other factors related to power and political care. This theory challenges nurse researchers, faculty, and clinicians to fully explicate the political, economic, social, and cultural values and the environmental factors influencing care in diverse groups, cultures, and institutions. Nursing students are always amazed to discover how politics and power are closely linked with gender and how social-structure factors exert tremendous influence within institutions, individuals, groups, and power alliances.

In the United States, power and politics are mainly embedded in economics, political and legal systems, technologies, and health care systems. In contrast, in many non-Western cultures, power and politics tend to be strongly linked with religion (or spirituality), kinship (extended family and group ties), and cultural values. Currently, in the United States' capitalistic system, a material goods and self-gain political ideology prevails. Accordingly, one finds American nurses emphasizing self-care ideologies and practices in nursing education and service. This emphasis fits Anglo-American values, but often fails to be congruent with many non-Western cultures (Leininger, 1991, 1994a, 1995). Such transcultural differences in the values and sources of politics and political factors need to be recognized and considered, to advance knowledge bearing on the humanistic and scientific dimensions of caring. Transcultural caring knowledge is also essential to understand differences and similarities in the power and politics of diverse organizational cultures. Thus, to transform nursing into a caring ideology and practice, nurses will benefit from studying the source and functions of power and politics in diverse cultures and institutions.

MEDICALIZATION: POWER AND POLITICS

One of the most difficult problems facing advancement of a caring ethos, practice, and institutional norms is the strong and dominant medical model that still pervades most hospitals and community health agencies, and many schools of nursing (Ashley, 1977; Leininger, 1994a). In the United States and in other countries, health institutions have been extensively medicalized; medical ideology, values, and practices are dominant forces and are buttressed by patriarchal medical leaders in the treating of pathological disease conditions. The medical model emphases are on curing diseases and pathologies, and relief of symptoms pervades the normative values, decisions, and operations of medical institutions. What is most needed in health and educational institutions is a pervasive and dominant focus on *caring as a way to know, understand, and help people*. This caring ethos and practice must be equated with or must offset the dominant medical model in order to meet current and future needs of consumers (Leininger, 1978, 1988a, 1988b, 1995). Now and in the future, human caring should become an explicit, central, and pervasive part of the healing and living environment of consumers in health and educational institutions. A caring ethos needs to be established as a power base with political strategies to *institutionalize caring* for the betterment of customers seeking health care and education. What people want most from health personnel, whether ill or well, is humanistic or scientific caring (Gaut, 1993; Leininger, 1976, 1988a, 1988b, 1992). Caring with a humanistic and transpersonal health perspective between client and nurse and between student and teacher can make a difference in the health and well-being of people (Boykin & Schoenhofen, 1993; Leininger, 1970, 1995; Watson, 1988). This caring perspective needs to become central to nursing education and human care services as the new and futuristic directions of the health reform movement.

For many years, nurses have been aware of medical power over nursing. Some power has been hegemonic in nature and such accounts have been documented in ethnographic, ethnonursing, and other qualitative studies (e.g., Ashley, 1977;

Leininger, 1970, 1994a, 1995; Street, 1992). The disparity of power in philosophy and practice between medicine and nursing needs to be reduced or redirected in order to make care viable and meaningful to clients. The use of research-based caring knowledge that is now available, such as presence, support, comfort, protection, touching, and many other kinds of transcultural caring expressions and practices, need to be explicitly and consciously taught and used in nursing education and service (Finn, 1993; Gaut, 1993; Leininger, 1988a, 1988b, 1991; Spangler, 1993; Stasiak, 1991; Wenger, 1992). Nurses are challenged to use these specific caring constructs in an explicit and planned way for the benefit of clients, students, faculty, and others, to provide culturally congruent and meaningful care services in nursing education and practice.

Currently, for many reasons, consumers in many places in the world are reestablishing their generic, folk, and naturalistic caring and healing modes. Some consumers are using generic or alternative holistic caring to support the "New Age Health Care Movement"—an indication that people are eager not only to use natural and familiar caring modes but to incorporate their spiritual, family, educational, political, religious, and other factors into healing and remaining well. Naturalistic modes of healing—touching, using cultural foods, massaging, and spiritual healing—are generic caring modes that are gradually being recognized and used with professional nursing care practices (Leininger, 1991, 1995). This is a good time and opportunity for nurses to blend generic and professional caring practices into all health care practices and into educational programs, to shift power from the medicalized disease treatment focus of curing to alternative caring, to help people use their familiar and alternative caring modes to remain well and prevent illnesses. Moreover, with the current emphasis on home care, primary care, and community-based services, the nurse with caring knowledge and skill is in the right position to integrate generic and professional care as an effective way to help people. This trend could well be one of the greatest and most powerful means to reform health care in meaningful and less costly ways. It could well shift nurses from the medicalized, institutionalized, and patriarchal dominated hospital ways to new ways of providing care that is meaningful and valued by diverse consumers. This strategy and similar ones need to be discussed in relation to planned ways to establish and institutionalize generic and professional nursing care.

Transcultural nursing knowledge from many cultures is another means or strategy to give power to nurses in caring processes and action modes. The Culture Care Theory supports the discovery of transcultural nursing knowledge (Leininger, 1989, 1991). This theory is invaluable to discover power and political thinking and actions related to consumers' needs and institutional practices. With the theory, existing political factors, worldview, language, and environmental contexts provide new insights and ways to care for people. Findings from the Culture Care Theory also help to discover women's naturalistic nurturance, their supportive and facilitative caring behaviors, and their roles in caring for people of different cultures. The theory explicitly helps to discover generic and professional caring *gender knowledge* from different cultures, as found in the work of Finn (1993), Gelazis (1993), and Spangler (1993), who identified political strategies and ways to provide culturally congruent nursing care norms, roles, standards, and practices in culture-specific ways. No longer should nurses keep invisible nursing's caring skills and knowledge. Such knowledge is a power source and a means to institute caring policies in nursing service and education. To deny caring services is unethical and weakens nurses' political power and significant contributions to humanity. Indeed, nurses have a moral obligation to teach and institutionalize male and female caring modes in the different environmental and cultural contexts in which they live and work.

CULTURES OF WOMEN AND MEN AS
CAREGIVERS: POLITICAL ASPECTS

In reflecting on the cultures of women and men as caregivers who have political power and perspectives, some interesting transcultural contrasts should be made explicit. Transculturally, in most societies, women have been the major caregivers. They have been involved in caring for family members throughout the life cycle. Often, the eldest daughter or the daughter still at home is expected to be the family caregiver (Brown, 1992; Leininger, 1991; Lindgren, 1993). Men have generally not been the principal caregivers unless they live in a matriarchal society in which the male offspring is expected to carry out female intergenerational norms and expectations. Because there are very few matriarchal cultures, such male caregiving family roles are limited. Women's caring roles, however, prevail transculturally and have throughout the history of homo sapiens. However, women's caring has not been made visible in public and social arenas. Moreover, women seldom show the political clout needed to make public policy related to major decisions in domestic or institutional health care. Nonetheless, women's caring roles have been extremely important to nurture, sustain, comfort, maintain, and support nuclear and extended family members throughout the life cycle. Most importantly, women in generic and professional caregiving roles have often prevented serious accidents, illnesses, and chronic conditions, and they have been the central caregivers in many Western and non-Western cultures (Brown, 1992; Leininger, 1988b, 1991). Women have often been caregivers to men; they have listened to, supported, and provided general counsel and nurturing to their husbands and other males with regard to their particular concerns and needs. It is, therefore, important to use women's care-giving power, and their generic and professional care knowledge, in framing and institutionalizing care policies and practices. It is also important to make known, in the public arenas, women's caregiving roles and especially professional nurses' role in maintaining health services.

STRATEGIES FOR NURSE CARE POWER AND POLITICAL DECISION

In the future, nurses need to give more attention to political strategies and power-based models that will make care visible and central to the discipline of nursing in institutional and noninstitutional contexts. Caring strategies are needed to make the public aware of the importance of care as a modality to nurture, heal, and help people. As nurses demonstrate quality of care, they need to make their nursing care skills known to those whom they serve. They need to publicize caring ways that show differences and similarities in different environmental care contexts, and the benefits of helping people to remain well. Nurses need to strategize and communicate the value of their work to legislators, influential politicians, key male and female leaders, and others who can support nurses' political efforts. In any institutions and cultures, political networking and fruitful connections with recognized leaders are essential to make caring an integral part of societal norms. The idea of marketing care in appropriate and respectful ways is important: care must be seen as a vital image of living, growing, and helping others. Political nursing strategies should be discussed and demonstrated in different caring contexts and documented with research methods such as narratives, audiovisual taping, ethnonursing phenomenology, and other methods. Nurses also need to share and apply their caring knowledge and skills in different settings. Most importantly, nurses should openly discuss and confront male-dominated, oppressive modes that limit women's full caring potential. Women nurses must emancipate themselves from working conditions and social systems that suppress the power and importance of caring. Dedication to human caring values and practices is essential as nurses work within multidisciplinary relationships and are responsible for teaching and mentoring students.

As nurses consider different models and theories that could help advance and substantiate care knowledge in practice and education, one of the models to be considered would be van Gennep's (1960) theoretical model on *rites of passage*. van Gennep, an anthropologist, was interested in the process of enculturation and how people in different cultures made changes or passages from one state to another. He postulated that there were rites of passage, consisting of the *rites of separation, transitional rites, and rites of incorporation* (van Gennep, 1960, p. 11). Each rite had shared patterns and practices that helped cultures move to important life-cycle changes. Nurses using van Gennep's rites of passage would be able to make a separation from the past medicine-dominated practices of nursing and to promote caring models of practice. As nurses move into the phase of transitional rites, they often experience uncertainty and marginal roles until the incorporation rites are established. Political strategies, policies, and group discussions are needed to help nurses move into the incorporation phase. When that phase is reached, nurses feel confident to act with an established caring philosophy; caring values and practices are central to their mode of functioning. Nurses would have also developed a strong caring ethos and would be politically active to retain this caring way of relating to others. Moreover, a collective image would be evident to consumers, who could then see the contributions of caring nurses in a society or culture. Hence, the challenge is to get caring institutionalized into all areas of nursing and within different cultures. Equally important, we must retain institutional caring policies and a caring philosophy. If such a caring philosophy prevails as a societal norm and agenda, one would predict less violence and abuse among humans, fewer killings, and, most of all, greater well-being.

Another important political strategy is to watch for the appropriate time to elect or get nurses with committed caring skills and expertise into key education and health institutions so that their ideas and practices can permeate the environment. To achieve this goal, nurses have to identify key leaders in advance, and then politically strategize to get them into key power positions. A collective political plan and action mode, buttressed by enthused, confident, and politically astute nurses, is needed to attain this goal. Positive responses and support for these care leaders and followers are essential to institutionalize caring and see caring outcomes.

Nurses also need to strategize in finding ways to use available research-based caring findings in nursing education and practice. It is especially important to use these findings in nursing practice and to uphold their positive benefits. Valentine's (1993) cogent work and research on the development of administrative and integrative ways to institutionalize caring in clinical practice is most important to consider. Her Clinical Incentive Program as an integrative process has benefits for hospital and nonhospital settings (Valentine, 1993, p. 331). Other research findings on care are now available from care researchers and need to be explicitly used in nursing practice as well as in nursing education (e.g., Boykin & Schoenhofer, 1993; Finn, 1993; Spangler, 1993).

The critical issues related to compensation for exquisite or competent caring practices continue to surface, especially when employers fail to value care.

Consumers ultimately will drive and influence most reimbursement for quality care. Politically, nurses and consumers, in partnership, need to demand quality care to prevent illnesses, hasten recovery, and provide healthy lifestyles. Nurses must demonstrate care outcomes to consumers in open, reaffirming, explicit, and confident ways. In addition, nurses need to join vigorously with consumers to seek funds for caring, research, education, and practice, so that care benefits can become institutionalized, valued, and protected in society. Recently, in Singapore, I witnessed how caring lifeways and practices, with prevention, health maintenance, and a planned public city agenda, were supported by public funds (Leininger, 1994b). The Singapore community programs are focused on caring lifestyles and prevention of illness. Such a caring and illness prevention model needs to be explored in different cultures and societies.

Today, nurses are increasingly aware of several established theories, and models, of research-based findings, and of practice examples that can serve to reinforce caring as the central and dominant focus of nursing. How to gain and use power and political strategies to make care central to nursing remains a stimulating and major challenge. The International Association of Human Caring, the Transcultural Nursing Society, the National League for Nursing, and the American Nurses Association all need to join forces to make care truly the focus of nursing in their political statements, and convention programs and in the public media. More politically committed care scholars and practitioners are needed to transform nursing education and practice.

I contend that the time is ripe for care to be an integral part of the New Age Movement worldwide. The New Age Movement is calling for cultural changes in the ways we view science, nursing, religion, politics, economics, and our spiritual and caring connectedness to people of diverse and similar cultures. The New Age Movement also indicates that our governing structures must become less fragmented, mechanistic, and impersonal. Most importantly, the New Age Movement needs and cries out for caring as an integral part of human relatedness, for healing, and for healthy ways of living, being, and dying. It also calls for actively institutionalized care in many societies so that care will be culturally transmitted to succeeding generations transculturally. Nursing and nurses need to enter and embrace this New Age Movement and politically make care knowledge and skill visibly and meaningful to humankind.

REFERENCES

Ashley, J. A. (1977). *Hospitals, paternalism, and the role of nursing*. New York: Teachers College Press.

Boykin, A., & Schoenhofer, S. (1993). *Nursing as caring: A model for transforming practice*. New York: National League for Nursing Press.

Brown, J. (1992). Lives of middle aged women. In V. Kern & J. Brown (Eds.). *In her prime: New views of middle aged women* (2nd Ed., pp. 17–30). Urbane: University of Illinois Press.

Finn, J. (1993). Caring in birthing: Experiences of professional nursing and generic care. In D. Gaut (Ed.), *A global agenda for caring* (pp. 63–80). New York: National League for Nursing Press.

Gaut, D. (Ed.). (1993). *A global agenda for caring*. New York: National League for Nursing Press.

Gelazis, R. (1993). Care: What it means to Lithuanian Americans. In D. Gaut (Ed.), *A global agenda for caring* (pp. 95–114). New York: National League for Nursing Press.

Kalisch, B., & Kalisch, P. (1982). *Politics of nursing*. Philadelphia: Lippincott.

Kottak, C. (1991). *Anthropology: The exploration of human diversity*. New York: McGraw-Hill.

Leininger, M. (1970). *Nursing and anthropology: Two worlds to blend*. New York: John Wiley & Sons. (Reprinted in 1994 by Greyden Press, Columbus, Ohio.)

Leininger, M. (1974). The leadership crisis in nursing: A critical problem and challenge. *Journal of Nursing Administration, 14*(2), 28–34.

Leininger, M. (1976). Caring: The essence and central focus on nursing. *American Nurses Foundation, Nursing Research Report, 12*(1).

Leininger, M. (1978). Political nursing: Essential for health and education systems of tomorrow. *Journal of Nursing Administration, 2*(3), 1–15.

Leininger, M. (1988a). *Care: An essential human need*. Detroit: Wayne State University Press. (Originally published in 1981 by Charles Slack, Thoroughfare, NJ.)

Leininger, M. (1988b). *Care: The essence of nursing*. Detroit: Wayne State University Press. (Originally published in 1984 by Charles Slack, Thoroughfare, NJ.)

Leininger, M. (1991). *Culture care diversity and universality: A theory of nursing*. New York: National League for Nursing Press.

Leininger, M. (1992). Culture care theory: A comparative global theory to advance human care nursing knowledge and practices. In D. Gaut (Ed.), *A global agenda for caring* (pp. 3–19). New York: National League for Nursing Press.

Leininger, M. (1994a). Tribes of nursing. *Journal of Transcultural Nursing, 6*(1), 18–22.

Leininger, M. (1994b, November 24). *Political leader in Singapore (personal communication)*.

Leininger, M. (1995). *Transcultural nursing: Concepts, theories, research, and practices*. New York/Columbus, OH: McGraw-Hill/Greyden Press.

Lindgren, C. (1993). The caregiver career. *Image: The Journal of Nursing Scholarship, 25*(3), 214–219.

Ray, M. (1989). The theory of bureaucratic caring for nursing practices in the organizational culture. *Nursing Administration Quarterly, 13*(2), 31–40.

Spangler, Z. (1993). Generic and professional care of Anglo-American and Philippine American nurses. In D. Gaut (Ed.), *A global agenda for caring* (pp. 47–62). New York: National League for Nursing Press.

Stasiak, D. (1991). Culture care theory with Mexican Americans in an urban context. In M. I.. Leininger (Ed.), *Culture care diversity and universality: A theory of nursing* (pp. 179–202). New York: National League for Nursing Press.

Street, A. F. (1992). *Inside nursing: A critical ethnography of clinical nursing practices.* Albany, NY: SUNY Press.

Valentine, K. (1993). Utilization of research on caring: Development of a nurse compensation system. In D. Gaut (Ed.), *A global agenda for caring* (pp. 329–347). New York: National League for Nursing Press.

van Gennep, A. (1960). *The rites of passage.* Chicago: University of Chicago Press.

Watson, J (1985). *Nursing: Human science and human care.* Norwalk, CT: Appleton-Century-Crofts.

Watson, J. (1988). *Nursing: Human science and human care: A theory of nursing.* New York: National League for Nursing Press.

Wenger, A. F. (1992). The Culture Care Theory and the Old Order Amish. In M L. Leininger (Ed.), *Culture care diversity and universality: A theory of nursing* (pp. 147–178). New York: National League for Nursing Press.

Williams, T. (1990). *Physical, cultural anthropology.* Englewood Cliffs, NJ: Prentice-Hall.

Part II

Power, Politics, and Public Policy:
The Practice Lens

6

Unleashing the Giant: The Politics of Women's Health Care

A. Lynne Wagner

HISTORICAL PERSPECTIVE

The care women receive in the medical system is molded by historical events, politics, religious dogma, and societal attitudes. Women have been leashed to a tradition of inadequate health care that, being deficient in understanding and respect, is inadequate in treatment and research. They have made gains to improve their health care, but continue to fight an age-old battle. Women's heritage is rich with examples of both victimization and accomplishments in health care.

Daughters of Time

Daughters of time,
in a wink you are gone,
but your stories stay strong.
With intuitive knowledge,
passed down by your mothers,
you have nurtured and bathed mankind.
Politics, economics, and fear of your secrets,

proved strong tides in the game of men.
You were swept away by the wrath of power.
Fear not as your spirit smolders in the ashes;
the magic of your presence is rekindled by your daughters.
The times are different,
but the battle is the same:
To claim rightful and equal place at man's side.

Women's new voice has begun to attract attention to the cause of improving their care and correcting injustices. Through storytelling, marching, lobbying, and forming support groups, they are combining their power for a more frontal attack for health care reform. Their targets are legislators who appropriate funds for research, doctors who diagnose and treat their diseases, drug and medical supply companies that develop products for women, and communities that interact daily with women living and coping with chronic and terminal illnesses. No study of today's women's demands for changes in their health care would be complete without understanding, through a historical perspective, that healing is power and power gets entrapped in the politics of daily living.

Early history portrays women as healers, as guardians who perpetuated secret formulas of birth, death, and living. Ancient mythology speaks of goddesses representing Good Mother Earth, who provided nourishment and healing magic (*Bulfinch's Mythology*, 1979). In Egypt, women healers had advanced knowledge of childbirth, abortion, and breast cancer (Boston Women's Health Book Collective, 1992). Greek and Roman mythology describes a plethora of goddesses graced with healing powers. Although it is not clear why and when women's influence declined, historians report that, by the time of Hippocrates (460 B.C.) and Aristotle (384 B.C.), women's representation in the healing arts was minimal and their status in society had been reduced to "assistant" or slave (Achterberg, 1991, p. 31).

Despite some evidence that the Church protected and respected women in abbeys during the 1300s, the stage was set by the tapestry of the male-dominated Christian Church to subjugate women's influence in society. Attempting to control the power of knowledge, the Church and the evolving scientific community excluded women from formal education. Knowledge gained outside the natural science of the Church was labeled magic or heresy, and was thought to be obtained from the devil. Women practicing the healing arts were accused of cohorting with the devil—the announced justification for witch trials, which resulted in an estimated 1 million female deaths over a 500-year period (1300–1700s) (Boston Women's Health Book Collective, 1992). The witch hunts diminished only as the Church's governing power waned in Europe, but the attitude of male dominance had a lasting impact on future generations (Dolan, Fitzpatrick, & Hermann, 1983; Donahue, 1985).

By the 17th century, the belief that women were spiritually deficient was expanded to include intellectual deficiency. It was believed that women were not only open to sensuality, but also motivated by illogical and irrational thinking and reactions (Chamberlain, 1981). The 19th-century philosopher Schopenhauer, whose views of women seem particularly apt for his time (n.d., pp. 64–67) wrote, "Women are childish, foolish, and shortsighted. . . . It is because women's reasoning powers are weaker that they show more sympathy for the unfortunate than men. . . . On the other hand, women are inferior to men in matters of justice, honesty, and conscientiousness. . . . They are to be admired only for their form."

Modern medical practices continue to be burdened by the misconceptions that women are incapable of understanding or coping and must be guided, shielded, and protected; that they are irrational and unable to report symptoms accurately; and that they are emotional and unstable, tending toward hypochondria. The established medical society has undermined the traditional healing wisdom of women by marketing health care as a commodity and eliminating the nurturing of women by women. Even in the 20th century, legislation was passed to outlaw midwifery, the last vestige of women's formal caring for women. Until nearly the 1970s, most women were treated by male doctors and gave birth in a hospital delivery room. The collective consequences of these events are still being felt to this day: a weakening of communication and of the special bonds between women, and a shifting of the power over women's health issues to paternalistic authority via the medicalization of normal events (Ehrenreich & English, 1981; Watson, 1994).

Women have not been silent and accommodating partners to these events. The pockets of explosion of women's fervor—for suffrage in the 1920s, for the feminist movement in the 1970s, and for better and more personalized health care in the 1990s—are direct reactions to this violation of basic rights and to a "second class" attitude toward women. Women have reported that doctors do not listen to them and sometimes do not believe them when they relate their symptoms. Knowledge is withheld or nonexistent. They encounter dishonesty and treatment without consent, are given incomplete information regarding risks (breast implants, DES, tamoxifen), and are given tranquilizers instead of resources to improve their coping. Treatment is often unnecessary, mutilating, and too severe for the problem (e.g., hysterectomies). Some women even report sexual abuse by health care providers (Corea, 1985; Dreifus, 1977; French, 1992; Smith, 1992).

Women now gather and share stories more openly. No longer will women suffer the injustices of a male-dominated system. As recently as 1969, little health information specifically for women was available (Boston Women's Health Book Collective, 1992). Women have fought for more partnership in their care, more respect, and more control, individually and as a gender group; they have been energized to create a resource for other women, not only to educate them, but to empower them to use the system to their advantage as well. Dreifus (1977) describes how the Women's Health Movement grew out of the larger Women's Movement in the 1970s and aimed to accomplish several goals: (a) changing public consciousness about women; (b) providing more health-related services; (c) changing attitudes about women in established health institutions; and (d) refocusing women's health care to include health education, prevention, and a sharing of skills and information.

Since the Women's Health Movement started in the 1970s, women have forced legislators, the Food and Drug Administration (FDA), doctors, religious leaders, and the public to reexamine and debate issues of abortion, childbirth practices, birth control, the dangers of freely prescribed hormones (the birth control pill, DES, and estrogen replacement therapy), the incomplete clinical trials and information on medications and devices (Flagyl, Dalkon shield), the unnecessary number of hysterectomies, the lack of health care among poor and rural women, the lack of female representation in health research (heart study programs), the narrowminded treatment of depression in women, and the mounting evidence that the medical system views male and female clients on different levels (Corea, 1985; Dreifus, 1977; Sanford & Donovan, 1984; Smith, 1992). These complaints have prompted hot debates and philosophical challenges. However, except in the case of abortion issues, many of these debates have stayed pocketed in small skirmishes and have effected only isolated changes in the health care system.

AN EXAMPLE OF CHANGE: THE POLITICS OF BREAST CANCER

On the other hand, the breast cancer battle has had a very dramatic impact. This campaign exemplifies the power of women to effect change. The epidemic proportions of this disease, which annually affects 180,000 women and kills 46,000, are being publicized daily in newspapers, talk shows, documentaries, advertisements, and books. Treatment and cure rates have not changed significantly in the past 50 years; medical care is often insensitive. Despite the fact that breast cancer destroys more lives than AIDS each year, research money for prevention and treatment has been sparse. Women meeting in small local groups have gathered a collective voice that is being heard now in Washington and is serving as a catalyst for change.

Of particular importance here is the National Breast Cancer Coalition, a grassroots advocacy effort created to focus national attention on the breast cancer epidemic. Formed in 1991, the Coalition encompasses 170 organizations representing several million patients, professionals, women, their families and friends. Their mission is to eradicate breast cancer by: advocating research into the cause, treatment, and cure for breast cancer through better funding; improving access to high-quality screening, diagnosis, treatment, and care for all women; and increasing the involvement and influence of women living with breast cancer. This grassroots advocacy has effected steady gains through the following efforts: (N. A. Ryan, NH Breast Cancer Coalition, personal communication, March 6, 1994):

1. *Legislative impact:*   The Coalition has steadily and successfully campaigned for increased research funding ($400 million in 1992 and $300 million in 1993) and the establishment of government-sponsored commissions, panels, departments, and agencies that specialize in women's health issues. The organization has spearheaded the passage of new laws, such as the Mammography Quality Standards Act of 1992.

2. *Grassroots mobilization and empowerment:*   The Coalition has been very successful in carrying out large grassroots signature campaigns, organizing rallies, and increasing the information available to women so they can become individually empowered in their interactions with the medical system.

3. *Media attention:*   The Coalition works closely with national and local media to keep breast cancer issues and concerns in front of policy makers and the public, through meetings with the President and Congressional leaders, rallies, and discussions of issues on talk shows and news analysis programs.

In the spirit of these pioneer women on the political scene, broadcaster Linda Ellerbee commented at the 1993 Washington rally, "We are not going to be good little girls. We are not going away, and we are not going to die politely" (Collins, 1994). When 2.6 million signatures were delivered to President Clinton, he promised more research money and announced a conference to begin drawing up a national plan. Under his health care plan, women will have increased benefits for breast exams and mammography (Clinton wants more, 1993).

The National Breast Cancer Coalition is supported by very active state coalitions whose members lobby, advocate, educate, and support on the local and national levels. Each state coalition sponsors one or two marches and rallies a year. The National Women's Health Network has joined forces with the Coalition, in addition to establishing its own front line of workers in the political battle of increasing awareness and policy surrounding breast cancer. The National Alliance Breast Cancer Organization (NABCO) and the American Cancer

Society serve as clearinghouses for information and resources. As a result, the Women's Health Initiative was formed in 1992. There are many local action groups. One sister group is the Women's Community Cancer Project, based in Cambridge, Massachusetts. This group is a volunteer organization created to make changes in current medical, social, and political approaches to cancers that affect women, with a special focus on environmental threats.

The government is not the only target in changing the system. Profit-making insurance companies also play a role in controlling the quality of health care through protocol setting, limitations on treatment and length of stays in hospitals, and policies of not insuring people for preexisting conditions. A study in the *New England Journal of Medicine* (Ayanian, Kohler, Abe, & Epstein, 1993) reports that uninsured patients and patients with Medicaid had more advanced disease when they sought health care and, therefore, had a lower survival rate than a group with private insurance who benefited from earlier screening and treatment. The authors concluded that lack of insurance coverage leads to poor outcomes because of the decreased access to screening and optimal treatment. With the present agitation for health care reform, the study supports the adoption of health care policies that encourage preventive health care and early diagnosis for all population segments.

Another controlling influence is the profit-making drug companies. Tamoxifen, which has been used for treating advanced breast cancer, is now being administered in large clinical trials, in hopes that it will prove effective in protecting women from breast cancer. Although the drug appears promising, it has reportedly not been proved safe, and many of the women taking it have not been informed of the possible side effects of blood clots, uterine cancer, liver cancer, or other unknown ramifications (Foreman, 1992d; Raloff, 1992, 1994).

The emotional and legal debates surrounding silicon breast implants are another illustration of how women's health suffers within the profit structures of the health industry. The silicon product had never undergone safety testing, the companies did not report problems that were recognized years before, and companies and physicians refused to believe women's concerns about and symptoms of side effects from the product. All of these factors combined to make this episode of deceit and fraud an emotional nightmare and physical trauma for women and their families (Foreman, 1992a, 1992b, 1992c; Understanding the debate, 1992; Vernaci, 1992). Medical supply companies and plastic surgeons had much to lose when silicon implants were implicated as unsafe and were removed from general use, but not as much as women whose health was impaired. The case for damage is so strong that several drug companies have settled a collective claim and will pay over $4 billion to the plaintiffs (Legal notice, 1994). The collective political action of women brought this problem to a head and challenged the "big guys." The effects are still being sorted out. Although some women are upset that the product is banned, many more women are angered and frightened by the deceit practiced against them.

Women and their families have pushed breast cancer into the public spotlight for high visibility. With the exception of AIDS, no other illness, especially a disease that primarily afflicts women, has commanded such coverage in lay and scientific media (Engelking, 1993). Brave and spirited women have put faces to the disease, personalizing it and challenging the stigma of being an imperfect female. Celebrities and public figures, such as Nancy Reagan, the women who are lobbying, the thousands of marchers who sport T-shirts and lapel buttons and exhibit personal courage have all awakened a public sense that this is not a pocketed disease that affects some strangers. Case histories, can get stale and be put out of mind. It takes women like Matuschka, a famous model, artist, and activist, to shock the public out of its complacency with her "Beauty Out of Damage" postmastectomy self-portrait, which was published in the *New York Times Magazine* (Ferraro, 1993). The impact was great enough for local newspapers to pick up on the article. The public responded both positively and negatively, but there was response. Matuschka said, "You can't look away anymore."

There is another political aspect to this tragedy: ongoing breast cancer research. Although new reports are appearing constantly, many are quite confusing and incomplete, which creates a dilemma both for women battling the disease and for doctors treating the women. Diet, alcohol consumption, exercise, antioxidants, environmental factors, genetic disposition, and estrogen exposure over a lifetime have all been reported to have some bearing on the disease. Two major organizations, the American Cancer Society and the National Institutes of Health, now debate the controversial issue of what age to start and how often to do mammography screening. Treatment modalities are not clear-cut, especially for early breast cancer, which leaves women and their doctors often playing a guessing game (Breast Cancer, 1988, Wallis, 1991).

Inaccurate research and misrepresentation of data add to the political turmoil that affects women's health care. On October 6, 1993, it was reported (Bass, 1993) that a mathematical error had been made in a major July 1993 study which had reassured women that a family history of breast cancer indicated only insignificant risk. The anxiety caused by such mistakes cannot be measured. It can also adversely affect a physician's screening plan for actually high-risk women.

More recently, questions have arisen out of reports of research fraud: who and what can a woman trust? In the landmark study of 20 years, which changed the choices and treatment of breast cancer dramatically by proving lumpectomies to be as lifesaving as mastectomies in many cases (Foreman, 1985), it was disclosed that some results had been falsified and, even worse, this information was covered up. Prestigious scientists have been dismissed during the outcry, but the damage has shaken the foundation of cancer research and treatment (Altman, 1994). Although the research outcomes appeared unchanged when adjusted for fraudulent data and the National Institutes of Health has stated that there was "no cause for concern" over the current treatment of the disease (New flaw reported, 1994, p. 1), doctors and patients alike are left bewildered and untrusting of all data on which protocols for treating illnesses are based.

The amassing of women, a giant on the move, has started to change the large organizations on the national and local front lines, but this change has not always filtered down to individuals. There are many women whose individual encounters with the disease and the medical system still evidence battle against inadequacies, insensitivity, and fragmentation of care. Out of this need have sprung support groups—women helping women to better cope with the disease, treatments, and their changing lives. Attitudes and grassroots policies are perhaps the most difficult to change, but individual women need to be empowered to advocate for themselves in doctors' offices. Their stories hold many clues to identifying the weaknesses and the strengths of the changing system. As I researched the history of women's health care and interviewed women who have health crises, I have come to value the dynamic connection between past and present, reflected in individual stories.

WOMEN'S STORIES OF THEIR ENCOUNTERS
WITH THE HEALTH CARE SYSTEM

I started my research by interviewing women with health problems, to discover common themes about how the medical system worked or did not work for them. My sample consisted of 11 Caucasian women, ages 32 to 62, one with arthritis, one with ovarian cancer, and nine with breast cancer. I captured the interviews through audio taping and note taking. Several positive and negative themes recurred in the women's perception of the care they received. Negative comments about the health care system described lack of information lack of support, insensitivity to client needs, and fragmentation of care (Table 6–1). The positive themes about the health care system stemmed from the women's active participation, coordination of care at comprehensive breast centers, and issues of advocacy (Table 6–2). Negative comments were more frequent; most of the women interviewed did not feel the health care system met their needs during their crises.

I am sharing with you summaries of several individual stories, for they give significant insight into the everyday politics in women's health care at the grassroots level. Along with their verbal narrations, I asked the women to submit an

Table 6–1 Negative Comments by Women about Their Interaction with the Health Care System

Themes	n[a]
Lack of information	11
Little or no support for family	11
Insensitivity to impact of disease	11
Fragmentation of care	9
Little or no support for woman	9
"Did not listen"	9
Had to demand second opinion	5
"Did not believe"	2
Did not fit into protocols	2

[a] Number of women (out of 11) who commented in each area.

Table 6–2 Positive Comments by Women about Their Interaction with the Health Care System

Themes	n[a]
Increased information with list of questions	11
Increased quality care with help of advocate	5
Coordination of care	2
Encouraged to get second opinion	2

[a] Number of women (out of 11) who commented in each area.

image that represented some aspect in their healing that would personalize their story. Several of those images are represented here. In addition to recording and analyzing each interview for its themes, I reacted to each story and expressed my interpretation of the themes in poetry. With the exception of one poem written posthumously, these poems have been verified by the women themselves for accuracy of interpretation.

Natalie

At 55 and menopausal, Natalie complained of vague symptoms: not feeling well, feeling bloated at times, excreting a watery vaginal discharge. After a battery of tests, no answers were found and her symptoms were dismissed as part of menopause. The symptoms persisted, but even with the additional onset of abdominal pain, Natalie was not taken seriously. She was treated casually for a vaginal infection and had no abatement of symptoms. For a year and a half, she searched in desperation for some doctor who would listen. Her records grew thicker with unfinding tests; a doctor told her it was all in her head. Finally, one doctor equated the vaginal discharge with ovarian cancer and offered an exploratory surgery. A ten-pound encapsulated ovarian tumor, the size of a honeydew melon, was discovered. After enduring months of chemotherapy and several more surgeries, Natilie died a year and a half after diagnosis, three years after her first symptoms appeared.

Natalie's Story: The Legacy

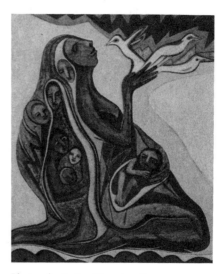

Because the system failed to listen,
did not believe the victim,
a funeral now to say goodbye,
ending one woman's chapter.
Tears flow to wash away the grief,
Clinging hugs comfort beating hearts.
The memories shared bond the living
*   spirit,*
And laughter heals the gap between
*   despair and hope.*
"Live on," says the Captain of the Day,
"For this is but a pause to recollect,
that death steals only the present, but
*   not the morrow.*
Do not let this death be for naught,
Take up the torch and march with force,
A warlike cry goes out
That future generations may live."

Photo of painting "Jamaica: Tomorrow,
Homage to Edna Manley," by Betty LaDuke.
Reproduced by permission of Betty LaDuke.

Diane

Diane is a 57-year-old woman with a history of cystic breast disease. When a lump showed up on her mammogram, no one was really concerned, but a biopsy proved the lump to be invasive lobular carcinoma. Because of her high risk of bilateral breast cancer, Diane decided to have a double mastectomy with reconstruction. Her story is riddled with complications, fragmentation of care, poor healing, and difficult psychosocial adjustments that she blames on medical incompetence, lack of educational and support information, and an insensitivity to her needs.

Diane's Story: Cradled in Healing Warmth

I bathe in being female,
Face uplifted to the sun,
Body caged, but floating free
In cleansing water, heated by my thoughts.
How ironic that such a private act
Should be a public show.
The politics of care
Have drained my senses dull,
Amputated with precision,
Then patched with body's flesh,
The only answer to give me life
When cancer invaded my breast.
The battle of my struggle proved the system weak
To offer preventive healing
In the wake of the invader's curse.
Care was uncoordinated,
At times delinquently unskilled,
To cause twice the mutilation,
Once of the body and then of the will.
What am I without a history,
Without a partnership in care?
Reduced to mechanism and robot stare,
Despite all odds, I heal;
The system can not reach me here.
I bathe in being female
And cleanse my spirit free.

Diana

Diana was 43 when she felt a lump in her breast. When cancer was diagnosed, her doctor recommended a mastectomy, but without sufficient explanation. Diana decided to have a lumpectomy. Three months later, another lump proved to be malignant and was followed by a lumpectomy, radiation, and chemotherapy. When a third lump was discovered a year later, Diana had a mastectomy with reconstruction. Despite her decision to stay in her local area for treatment so she could be with family and friends, she speaks of emptiness and loneliness for which she was not prepared. These feelings were augmented by additional surprises, such as her sudden symptomatic menopause and other side effects of her chemotherapy and surgery.

Diana's Story: Emptiness

The fullness of my life drained out
through the incision across my chest.
I did not realize how much I harbored there,
until I felt the emptiness.
More than the weight I missed,
but rather the richness of life's milk.
Who am I without this piece of flesh?
How like a room without its furniture,
a poverty felt between the boundaries of the walls.
Lacking information, I could not fill the gap.
Slowly now I'm finding ways to replenish,
a new and different kind of space.
I tell you my story to help you understand.
When you mutilate the next woman
with the thought of saving lives,
know your prognosis does little good,
without empowering her as team mate.
Healing comes in many forms,
that are not reflected in the scars.
You must help me heal my spirit,
along with the physical pain.
We then will celebrate victory together,
and life won't be so empty hearted.

Marcia

Marcia, a 56-year-old woman diagnosed with infiltrating intraductal carcinoma, had a mastectomy after a two-month delay due to scheduling problems. Waiting for lymph node results, she experienced poor communication. Married, with grown children, she is raising two grandchildren. Her sole reason for living is for her family, and her fears of letting them down were never addressed in her recovery. Her story exemplifies the system's insensitivity to individual needs, the indecisiveness of medical protocol, and the lack of support for the woman and her family.

Marcia's Story:
Where Is the Caring?

*I called the doctor today and was put on
  hold,*
Left to listen to the echo of my breath.
Where is the caring?
*I had a doctor's appointment today and
  sat for an hour,*
Background music and Ladies' Home
  Journal *padded empty time.*
Where is the caring?
*Exam complete, "You're fine until next
  visit," says he,*
*Not a chance to tell him how I hurt
  inside.*
Where is the caring?
*He listened to my heart, palpated my
  scars,*
*But never heard my grandchildren's
  fears.*
Where is the caring?
*Breast gone. Hair gone. Tired. How
  can I look fine?*
*Through what special glasses is he
  looking at me?*
Where is the caring?

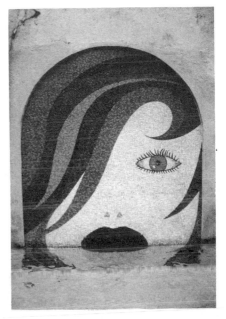

Modern mosaic of woman's face, photo taken
by A. Lynne Wanger in Tremezzo, Italy.

Lauren

Lauren is a 48-year-old postmenopausal woman who had a 13–14-year history of a benign lump that appeared and disappeared around her menstrual cycles. It suddenly became inflamed and, on biopsy, was discovered to be a 3A invasive carcinoma. She was treated with chemotherapy, followed by a mastectomy, radiation, and a second course of very aggressive chemotherapy. As a result of the chemotherapy, she has developed severe osteoporosis and a thyroid tumor. She states, "I have to advocate for myself. I feel I have to find answers in the literature myself. No one told me to increase my calcium during chemotherapy. I had to constantly remind them that when they changed my appointments due to their busyness, they caused a strain on my busy schedule. I felt as though they had no respect for me. I was constantly amazed at the lack of new medical knowledge in the breast cancer arena." Lauren really felt her whole treatment schedule was "an experiment" and the doctors themselves were learning the long-term effects of aggressive chemotherapy. No one empowered her to use her own resources.

Lauren's Story: The Battle Lines

War had been declared
and I formed my lines of battle.
Alliances came forward to march with me,
most untested by prior crises,
But cancer appeared our common enemy.
The first were my doctors, experienced generals.
They planned, "We'll poison, then cut him out."
So I lost my hair and flesh with little hope.
To boost our chances, one general said in expertise,
"We'll burn him out."
"At what expense?" said I.
"Some red skin and tiredness, like after any battle."
So the war raged for six more weeks,
Small skirmishes each day at the battlefield,
And the losses took their toll,
Not as obvious as the scars of the first battle,
But tiredness robbed me of my job.
Still my generals plotted at their separate planning tables,
As the enemy laughed from my nodes.
"We saved the worst till last;
we'll flush him out with special poison."
Numbed by now with battle fatigue,
I did not question my advisors.
So I endured the ravages of my last stand
With nausea, hair loss, and disassociation from self.
I understand to fight well and kill,
A soldier must just react, not think.
But my generals forgot to tell me, I also needed faith.
I was so intent in the Board Room,
I never looked up to see my second line of defense,
My footsoldiers who had marched with me.
They never faltered in driving me to battle each day,
or in supporting the baldheaded mother.
The system of warfare had failed us all,

So impersonal and secretive in their decisions.
They planned the attacks with incomplete information.
We battled for balance with little preparation.
Now united, my footsoldiers and I claim victory in our game of life.

Annette

Annette is a 32-year-old, unmarried, cosmetic makeup artist and an athlete. Her story challenges the medical system and policy makers to reexamine genetic influences of breast cancer and treatment protocols. With a family history of her mother and aunt both having had breast cancer at an early age, Annette, at age 31, battled with her HMO to waive its protocol (based on age) for who is eligible to receive mammograms. She insisted that she needed to start surveillance early. Finally winning, she had a mammogram done that year, which proved normal and served as a base-line for comparison a year later, when her second mammogram showed microcalcifications. A biopsy indicated an intraductal carcinoma in situ. She found the medical world did not really know how to treat her early cancer at such a young age, but strongly suggested a mastectomy as a prophylactic measure against reoccurrence. Once diagnosed, the system did respond to Annette in a positive, supportive way, perhaps due to her youth and her self-confidence. The following poems address two aspects of her story.

Annette's Story: So Much for Protocol

I am angry that history repeats
with still no hope of cure,
Twenty-five years have passed
since cancer claimed mother and aunt,
And now the offspring encounters similar fate
Amidst fraudulent research of family genes.
I can't believe that in all these years
with so many lives at stake,
that policy makers have failed to provide
answers to prevent a most deadly disease.
Don't be so rigid in hearing my pleas.
Mutilating treatment remains the best weapon,
Difficult at age 32.
Unmarried, I stand a marked woman,
Beauty scarred in society's eyes.

But in my quest for a full life,
I join the marching force,
and demand that the system respond
to the call of the wild women, dying and brave,
more research, more answers, more care,
so the next generation won't fall.

Annette's Story: Empowerment

The system worked for me,
caring hands, coordinating minds,
looking for answers, making no promises,
empowering me to find my way,
through maze of choices,
lifting up my resources,
to support me in my weakness,
to magnify my strengths.
Reduced to a bundle of fears,
confused and feeling alone,
the "Why me" dissolved into "Let's go,
I'm ready, world, to take you on."

Diane

Diane is a 48-year-old woman and nurse who had been followed closely over an 18-month period for a suspicious mammogram. Changes prompted a biopsy, which proved positive. Although Diane had decided to have a lumpectomy, the day before her scheduled surgery, the radiologist informed her that the cell constellation did not appear to be treatable with radiation follow-up. Therefore, without time to process, Diane found herself in surgery the next day for a mastectomy, which was followed by chemotherapy. She complained angrily about the lack of coordination and communication in her care between her caregivers. Because she felt fragmented, she had little control over her decisions and support systems. One ramification of this distress was her relationship with her husband. Neither she nor he was prepared for her severe menopausal symptoms brought on by the chemotherapy or for the adjustments in their intimacy. Far more devastating than the disease process and treatment was her husband's announcement that he wanted twin beds, which added to her intense loneliness and alienation of self.

Diane's Story: Fragmentation

*My double-breasted chest, reduced to
one.
My double bed is split in two.
My life is shattered by this singleness,
Fragmentation separates my body from
my heart.
Can't he understand I have only lost
one part?
Society paints his fantasy of perfect
mate.
My doctors unconcerned about our fate.
I am alone at the height of my need,
No breast, no hair, no more seed.*

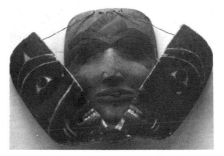

Transformation mask, Haida, 19th c. (American Museum of Natural History, New York); source: Moyers, B. (1993). *Healing and the Mind*. New York: Doubleday, p. 5, color plates. Neg. No. 2A12617, Courtesy of Department Library Services, American Museum of Natural History.

These are but a few examples of the stories being told, and my humanness is touched by each of them. No matter how many gains are made in the political arena for improved health care of women, until it has filtered down to each individual, no victory is complete. These women's stories are not meant for the history books, but for active change. I asked one woman why she was marching in Boston when she was so sick. She told me that she feels a little like Don Quixote. Her mother and grandmother had both died at an early age of breast cancer. She wants her daughter to have a chance to survive the trauma and the curse of this dread disease. She recited to me the lyrics of "The Impossible Dream," a song that most of us know well and which she is guided in her quest for better policy making, better research at the top, and more accepting attitudes at the local level to provide a better future for those who survive.

Sara died a month ago. Her 16-year-old daughter now carries the burden and the torch. The complex mixture of hopelessness and future dreams being played out in the present is embodied in this one story that captures the spirit of all the stories I have heard. Listen to those close and not so close to you, look deeply into the complex dimension of women's struggles, and you too will know more about the changing impact of health care for women.

REFERENCES

Achterberg, J. (1991). *Woman as healer*. Boston: Shambhala.

Altman, L. K. (1994, March 15). Cancer study used false data. *International Herald Tribune*, p. 1.

Ayanain, J., Kohler, B., Abe, T., & Epstein, A. (1993). The relationship between health insurance coverage and clinical outcomes among women with breast cancer. *New England Journal of Medicine, 329*(5), 326–331.

Bass, A. (1993, October 6). Cancer study error found. *Boston Globe*, pp. 1, 18.

Breast cancer: Early decisions. (1988, March). *Harvard Medical School Health Letter*, pp. 1–4.

Boston Women's Health Book Collective. (1992). *The new our bodies, ourselves*. New York: Simon & Schuster.

Bulfinch's mythology. (1979). New York: Crown Publishers.

Chamberlain, M. (1981). *Old wives' tales: Their history, remedies, and spells*. London: Virago Press.

Clinton wants more breast cancer study. (1993, October 19). *Boston Globe*, p. 1.

Collins, P. (1994, Winter). In Washington, D.C., for signature drive. *NH Breast Cancer Coalition Newsletter: Raising Our Voices*, pp. 1–2.

Corea, G. (1985). *The hidden malpractice: How American medicine mistreats women*. New York: Harper & Row.

Dolan, J., Fitzpatrick, M. L., & Hermann, E. K. (1983). *Nursing in society: A historical perspective* (15th ed.). Philadelphia: Saunders.

Donahue, M. P. (1985). *Nursing: The finest art (An illustrated history)*. St. Louis: Mosby.

Dreifus, C. (Ed.). (1978). *Seizing our bodies: The politics of women's health*. New York: Random House.

Ehrenreich, B., & English, D. (1978). *For her own good: 150 years of experts' advice to women*. New York: Doubleday.

Engelking, C. (1993). The breast cancer movement: Playing our part. *Innovations in Oncology Nursing, 9*(4), p 1.

Ferraro, S. (1993, August 15). You can't look away anymore: The anguished politics of breast cancer. *New York Times Magazine*, pp. 24–27.

Foreman, J. (1985, March 14). Study backs less surgery in breast cancer. *Boston Globe*, pp. 1, 10.

Foreman, J. (1992a, January 7). FDA moratorium on breast implants. *Boston Globe*, pp. 1, 14.

Foreman, J. (1992b, January 13). Implants: Is uninformed consent a woman's right? *Boston Globe*, pp. 1, 29.

Foreman, J. (1992c, January 19). Long-term safety was concern of researchers for implant maker. *Boston Globe*, p. 23.

Foreman, J. (1992d, April 29). US to begin a wide test of breast cancer drug. *Boston Globe*, pp. 1, 12.

French, M. (1992). *The war against women*. New York: Ballantine Books.

Legal notice. (1994, April 26). All persons who have ever had breast implants. *USA Today*, p. 2.

Moyers, B. (1993). *Healing and the mind*. New York: Doubleday.

New flaw reported in cancer studies. (1994, March 30). *Boston Globe*, p. 1.

Raloff, J. (1992, November 28). Tamoxifen and informed consent dissent. *Science News*, pp. 378–380.

Raloff, J. (1994, February 26). Studies spark new tamoxifen controversy. *Science News*, p. 133.

Schopenhauer: Essays of Schopenhauer. (no date). Translated by Mrs. Rudolf Dircks. London: Walter Scott, Ltd.

Smith, J. M. (1992). *Women and doctors*. New York: Dell.

Understanding the debate over breast implants. (1992, February). *NAACOG Newsletter*, pp. 1, 6–8.

Vernaci, R. L. (1992, February 25). FDA will ask for safety records from all breast implant makers. *Boston Globe*, p. 6.

Wallis, C. (1991, January 14). A puzzling plague. *Time*, pp. 48–55.

Watson, J. (1994). The moral failure of the patriarchy. In E. C. Hein & M. J. Nicholson (Eds.), *Contemporary leadership behavior*. Philadelphia: Lippincott.

7

Caring at the Crossroads: The Need for an Interpretive Strategy

Patricia Farrell
Gary Nuttall

Increasingly, nurse administrators have become explicitly focused on the core value of caring and what caring means, particularly in this time of economic restraint and health care reform. One of the major themes in the literature is the fit of caring and its holistic, humanistic perspective with the business model of management and its primarily empirical orientation. The humanistic approach and the empirical approach are viewed as fundamentally in conflict with regard to their basic value assumptions (e.g., Brenner & Marz, 1986; Brown, 1991; Cronkhite, 1992; Lumby & Duffield, 1993; Miller, 1987; Mowinski Jennings, 1987; Nyberg, 1993; Ray, 1987). Nurse administrators are caught with one foot in each view and are struggling with strategies to resolve the apparent conflict. Various strategies have been proposed, for example: collective lobbying with government for a care agenda (Gordon, 1991); using alternative care delivery models and leading-edge management techniques to enhance staff nurse empowerment (Ameigh & Billet, 1992; Porter O'Grady, 1992; Wells, 1993); and identifying and using caring behaviors in nursing management (Duffy, 1993; Dunham, 1989; Muller, 1993; Nyberg, 1989).

We propose a strategy that is different from those identified in the literature. We contend that North America is in the midst of an unprecedented values shift, and that the explicit assumption of a conflict between humanistic and empirical values must be challenged. In this chapter, we illustrate how the identification of overlap in the values of nurse leaders and of nurses in direct care at the unit level is a necessary strategy prior to the adoption of any alternative management approaches or techniques. We also challenge the implicit assumption that caring for the system—for example, by experimenting with new management approaches—is synonymous with caring for the patient or client. Finally, we suggest how caring can be a major force in bridging seemingly conflicting values.

Prior to addressing these issues, we provide a description of what we mean by values. We also highlight the methodology used in our values research projects, which differs from traditional approaches in distinguishing opinions and attitudes from more deeply held values.

RESEARCH FRAMEWORK AND METHODOLOGY

We have been developing our framework and methodology to obtain data on values for several years. In the health sector, our research with nurses has included staff nurses and administrators in both hospital and community organizations, including an overall database on values from 26,800 nurses (Nuttall, Farrell, Nuttall, & Nuttall, 1994; Nuttall & Nuttall, 1992; Nuttall, Nuttall, & Farrell, 1993, 1994).

Historically, studies of organizations and their members have been framed as goal-attainment and systems studies (e.g., Davies, 1988; Eilon, 1990), organizational behavioral studies (e.g., Miles & Randolph, 1980; Miller & Friesen, 1980; Shrivastava & Mitroff, 1982), and studies of the culture of organizations (e.g., Schein, 1984; Wilkins & Ouchi, 1983). Goal-attainment, systems, and organizational behavior studies are mainly not concerned with the study of individual and group values within the organization. Organizational culture studies, however, assume that values are inherent in the culture of the organization and are an essential focus for research.

Typical methodologies employed in studies of organizational culture include both traditional empirical approaches, such as the use of questionnaires and organizational audits (developed by researchers with their own value sets about what constitutes values and culture), and traditional anthropologic approaches via participant observation. Participant observation is guided by the principle that immersion in the culture of the organization, and dialogue with and observation of informants, will reveal that culture and its values (Schein, 1990).

We assume that individuals and groups, if provided with a process, can identify their own values. Such a process is critical to avoid what we now call the artifact of "learned values." This artifact results when the researcher and participant engage in values clarification exercises. The participant normally provides the researcher with a learned response that supports the group's learned beliefs (Schein, 1984). In the case of health care, this artifact frequently appears as an acceptable context within a group that supports that group's health care delivery system.

The artifact of learned values also frequently appears when large polls of public opinion are conducted. Depending on the questions asked, the results will reveal one and ignore other forms of values (Hall, 1981). Here is where we have distinguished between opinion or attitude (one form of values) and values of a higher priority that may not be acceptable for the individual or group to express. Verbally expressed opinions and attitudes tend to be more superficial—what the reference group wants to hear and what the participants want it to hear.

Participants and researchers belong to many different reference groups and may espouse opinions and attitudes reflective of any one or many of these groups. Figure 7–1 illustrates individuals and groups within organizations, and

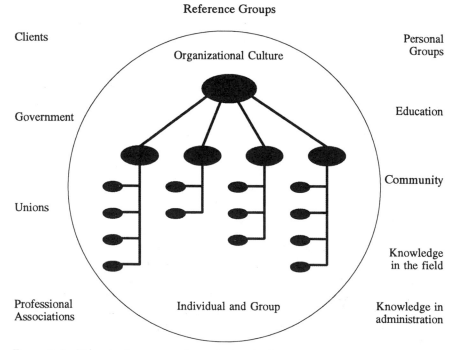

Figure 7–1   Values in the context of organizational culture.

a few of their many reference groups. Our research indicates that the values of more and more of these reference groups are gaining a higher priority for nurses within their employment settings.

Higher-priority values, as opposed to the more superficial values of attitude and opinion, are deeply held and provide a more solid basis for action than do attitudes and opinions. Higher-priority values may not easily be verbally expressed, or they may be expressed in abstract terms or symbols that are not easily analyzed for their direct effects on behavior (Trice, 1993). Yet, these values will direct behavior. For example, the concept "staffing" was a symbol traditionally used by nurses to describe a process that ensures the availability of appropriately trained and effective colleagues who can work well together. More recently, our research reveals that the concept of staffing is now symbolizing patient and client safety as well as the loss of nursing jobs (Aylward & Nuttall, 1994). It has taken on a new meaning that is a more deeply held, higher-priority value than that of working with competent colleagues. The process or methodology that we use in identifying the deeper values, even when the traditional learned values have been expressed, is designed to cut through the layers of attitudes and opinions expressed by individuals. It is designed to identify the core, higher-priority, and deeply held values of the group. Briefly, we use the following process:

1. Focus groups, comprised of members of the group or organization, tell us what issues are important to them in their organization. The research variables are derived from each focus group rather than from the researchers. By rotating the chairperson role within each group, the group is consistently turned inward, rather than outward to a focus group leader or moderator.

2. The issues from the focus groups are formatted into: (a) questionnaires that are mailed to every member of the organization; (b) one-on-one interviews in person and by telephone; and (c) additional focus groups. These methods are used to seek agreement on whether the identified issues are recognized as issues for members, and to ascertain a cross-similarity of meaning between subgroups such as different institutions. Ascertaining a cross-similarity of meaning enables us to better describe the issues of interest in terms that all participants will understand.

3. The results of these surveys, interviews, and focus groups are presented to different focus groups within the organization, to tell us the stories of the issues. Are the issues recognizable as exemplars? Do they "feel right"? What symbols emerge? The goal is to determine the underlying values rather than the "talk of the moment."

4. The issues and symbols are entered into the qualitative computer program especially developed for our research. The program enables us not only to search the data within the organization under study, but also to

search for patterns in our entire data set, which is comprised of many studies, both nursing and non-nursing.

5.   New patterns or perplexing and unusual combinations of patterns are next discussed, using telephone interviews, with a sample of members within the organization. Here, in the interests of further refinement, we continue to ask questions to build context around new or unusual patterns. We ask: How is this pattern exemplified in professional nursing practice?

6.   The issues are refined into precise statements of values that are formatted into questionnaires and mailed to members for their agreement, disagreement, or uncertainty. If necessary, we will use more focus groups in situations where there are seemingly conflicting values. In other words, we can describe situations where one value takes a higher priority over another, as in the staffing example cited earlier.

Only when we have proceeded through this process do we assume we have information about the values of a group—information that will feel right, at the "gut" level, to its members. This process may suggest a Delphi methodology (Linstone & Turoff, 1975). Our process is similar to the Delphi, but instead of using a panel of expert informants, we use many groups and different individuals, as well as the entire membership, at various times in the process. Also, we do not build intellectual consensus through iterative phases as does the Delphi. In fact, we may end up with multiple "truths," all of which feel right to members. These truths may have increased or decreased priority over various contexts.

Also, unlike the Delphi, we continuously overlay participants' responses on our larger data set, which provides a kind of societal backdrop for the study of the moment. Currently, our data set contains values from over 500,000 individuals who have participated in our research. Our program enables us to ask questions such as: Is this value, held by nurses, also held by physicians, or administrators, or teenagers? We can also ask: What are the symbols of this value, and do the symbols differ across groups? In this way, we have been able to identify what we referred to earlier as an unprecedented values shift.

UNPRECEDENTED VALUES SHIFT

When comparing our data sets retrospectively, in response to some curious patterns that repeated in our findings since 1990, we identified (tentatively labeled, in 1990) an ideological values group and a new pragmatic values group. We identified a shift from ideological to pragmatic values.

The ideological values group is characterized by a set of beliefs in the system and a sense of justice or "moral" rightness in connection with these beliefs. There is a profile of "correct" behavior espoused by this group. The ideological values group is actually comprised of two age groups: (a) an older group of about age 60 and above and (b) a group of 1960s people who are about ages 30 to 50 and slightly above. The two groups generally have different ideologies, as we will illustrate; however, they consistently fit the ideological values characteristics cited above. In our research, we define ideology as: the accepted culture of the organization; the way things are done; the normal course that decision making follows; the accepted artifacts of correctness; and beliefs that lead to success. In the words of Feuer (1975), ideology is the "outcome of social circumpressures . . . it takes philosophy and reduces it to the lowest common social denominator . . . it closes the door to search and doubt" (p. 188).

The pragmatic values group, only recently, is being partially described in the popular press as "Generation X." Currently, the press writers have correctly identified a new values set, but are trying to explain this set ideologically. For example, Generation X frequently is referred to as having no morals, or as behaving irresponsibly. We, as researchers engaged in values research, have characterized the new, pragmatic values group as having a "whatever works" approach. People in the pragmatic values group are not guided by ideology and will use ideology only if it is pragmatic to do so. We illustrate with the following true story of a man aged 63 years; a 40-year-old man; and a 22-year old man. The ideological values and pragmatic responses are labeled. The use of several exploratory responses to an issue is characteristic of people in the pragmatic values group.

> One day, as I was impatiently waiting, for some time, to give a younger colleague a ride home, I went over to a coke machine and deposited my money to get a coke. I lost my last coin in the machine. As I was trying to get my money back, an older man came along and saw my problem. He said:
>
> "They don't make them the way they used to." [ideological value]
>
> We chatted about this and about how organizations must work to improve and how work attitudes should improve. He then said:
>
> "If you go down the hall to the office, you can fill out a chit and they will send your money back to you."
>
> Not wanting to be bothered with this, I continued to manipulate the machine. Another man came over. This man looked to be in his late 30s or 40s. He said:
>
> "Having trouble with the machine, eh? Those damn machines! They're designed that way!" [ideological value]
>
> I asked him to help, so he gave the machine a kick and a shove. When that didn't help, I told him that I had been told I could go down the hall and

fill out a chit to get my money back. He reacted rather negatively to this option and left. By now I was getting interested in this natural experiment unfolding before me. Finally, after a considerable wait, my younger colleague came along and asked me if I was ready to go. I said:

"Wait a minute. I've lost my money in the Coke machine."

My colleague said:

"So? Do you need some money?" [pragmatic response]

I replied:

"No. It's not the money. It's the principle of the thing. I want it back from the machine."

My colleague responded:

"Okay. I have things to do right now. I'll just go on with my friend if you want to stay and deal with this machine." [pragmatic response]

I indignantly replied:

"Hold on! I've waited for you all this time. Now you can just wait until I get my money out of this machine and, don't forget, you may need a ride from me in the future."

At this point, my colleague shrugged his shoulders and went over and gave the machine a light jiggle back and forth and my money came out! I said:

"That's amazing. What would you have done if that hadn't worked?"

He replied:

"If that doesn't work, and if for some reason you need the money, I've heard that if you lay the machine on its face you can dismantle part of it and get your money." [pragmatic response]

Note the pattern here. The older man had an ideological belief that problems do occur with organizations and with workers, but there is provision and there are trends in the system to take care of these problems. He is willing to wait. The "1960s" person also had an ideological belief that the system was designed to "get" us. He could become violent against the system and was unwilling to wait. The new pragmatic values group person would use whatever works, even an ideological solution such as going down the hall and filling out a chit, if it made sense according to his information and values. The pragmatic values group doesn't worry about traditional system beliefs as much as does the ideological group. Members of the pragmatic values group simply want to survive in the most effective manner. If the system isn't making sense, they find their own multiple solutions or they withdraw. Also, they can shift quickly from one solution to another, leaving a confused ideologue asking, "Just where do they stand?"

Nurses in our current studies represent both values groups, and it is extremely frustrating for nurse administrators, who currently are mostly in the ideological group, to "manage" nurses in the pragmatic group. We frequently hear, "I don't know where these new graduates are coming from! They don't seem to care! What [ideology] are they being taught in school or in their homes?" We have found that nurse administrators need new skills in management, as is recommended in the literature, but not because of a conflict in values. Rather, they need processes to reveal the values, with all of their multiple truths (pragmatic, ideological, and so forth), and strategies to directly incorporate these values into their management decision-making systems and behaviors. In this way, the organization or system can become a professional system for care that is more synonymous with caring for the patient or client.

CARING FOR THE SYSTEM OR CARING FOR THE PATIENT AND CLIENT?

We have suggested that, by identifying and incorporating values into administrative decisions, a more caring and cared-for system will evolve: a system that will include both the humanistic truths and the empirical truths. In our recent work, we have gained some further insight into a values phenomenon that is peculiar only to nurses. This phenomenon is peculiar to nurses because of their core value of caring as well as how they are valued by others. We have discovered that no matter how cumbersome or inappropriate new management technologies are, nurses will attempt to make them work. They will treat them as "sick" and in need of care. For example, when computer systems were established in nursing units in several hospitals, traditional surveys of the impact on nurses revealed that, although there were problems with the implementation of the change, nurses were managing the change and finding it exciting and challenging. These findings are an example of what we define as superficial values or truths. Our cultural research data revealed another, more deeply held value. Nurses believed that the current computer systems would not save them time or benefit them in any real way. Rather, these systems were something they could do nothing about; the decision for implementation had already been made by higher authorities, and the best the nurses could do was to try to make things better. They were caring for the system in much the same way they cared for their patients and clients. The following data from our studies provide an illustration:

> The program for learning about computers is very inefficient and intimidating. It takes time away from our patients. They are a pain in the neck, but computers are here to stay in our life. I guess we will get used to them.

It's the way of the future, but it's introduction to our hospital was abysmal and wasted a lot of time and money . . . eventually, I guess they will succeed.

They are a reality, though not dependable. They triple our workload.

It's the pits for nurses. It takes us away from our patients, wastes paper and money. It's good for medical records, though.

I could write a thesis on this! Administrators failed nurses by introducing a system that doesn't work. Now we nurses are making it work but it is a headache, and expensive to implement.

This core value of caring for the system has become a real challenge in this time of health care reform. Nurses currently are caring for new systems of staffing and new methods of care delivery, as well as struggling to care for patients and clients within these contexts. Because, in many cases, they cannot cope (pragmatically) or care (ideologically or pragmatically), nurses are sinking into apathy. How, then, is caring demonstrated at the unit level, or the immediate work site?

CARING IN THE CONTEXT OF THE IMMEDIATE WORKPLACE

Frequently, we hear nurse administrators despair that staff nurses don't have a larger view of the organization, or a broader view of directions in the profession itself. This notion that staff nurses have a limited view frustrates nurse administrators who are attempting to ensure a competent professional staff that is responsive to the larger, systemwide economic issues, and thus flexible enough to permit needed reforms or change within the organization. The staff nurses, in our research, do have these larger, systemwide views. However, these views frequently are not expressed in surveys or interviews and may even be masked because of a higher-priority, deeply held value: valuing the immediate work site.

This valuing of the immediate work site was identified as we compared our qualitative and quantitative data sets. Symbols of the immediate work site, such as the nature of nurse and physician colleagues, clustered together differently than did the general descriptions of nurses and physicians. We took this finding to focus groups and asked them to explore the question: "When I go to work, I am thinking _____ ." This process helped us to determine the priority of the valuing of the work site.

Staff nurses deeply value their work site, the smaller unit where they work. When they go to work, they are thinking of the availability of competent colleagues, their particular patient assignment, and whether they will be able to cope with the assignment. Following are some illustrations from our research.

When I go to work, I am thinking that I hope no one called in sick. How busy will the unit be? What will my assignment be?

What kind of shift will I have? Let there be enough good staff. Can I make a difference for my patients and their families?

I hope my energy lasts all day. Who will I care for and who is working with me?

Also, although nurses may be critical of physicians as a group, they will hesitate to criticize physicians on their unit. Even when a physician is known to be difficult, they will identify him or her as part of a sick system and employ cover-up strategies. Following are data from our research illustrative of nurses' valuing of physicians generally and of physicians at their immediate work site:

Doctors are arrogant and don't communicate. On our ward they are professional.

Doctors are dictorial, self-serving, and overpaid. They are great on our unit.

This valuing of one's own unit and its physicians has implications for decision-making systems in organizations. The ideological value is that physicians make decisions in the medical world and nurses care by implementing these decisions. To destroy the medical decision system and build a nursing decision system—as is required, for example, in models of nurse-managed care—is symbolic of not caring from the point of view of the ideological values group. However, it is a good example of caring to the pragmatic values group. Nurses in the pragmatic values group want to redesign the decision-making system for the good of the health care delivery system. If they cannot redesign from a perspective that is effective and efficient for the working unit, they will become militant or apathetic, as our data reveal. An effective working unit, to the pragmatic values group, is comprised of nurses who have the legitimate authority to make decisions that will improve the quality and cost-effectiveness of health care.

In addition to implications for decision-making systems, the valuing of one's own unit has implications for management practices. How do nurses, at the unit level, value their nurse administrators? We have found that there is a gap between nurses and their nursing leaders that is expressed as a strongly held value.

THE GAP BETWEEN NURSES AND
THEIR NURSING LEADERS

Staff nurses incorporate their immediate supervisors (for example, head nurses) into their work site and assess the competence of these managers as they do that of any other peer colleague. However, one level removed from the immediate work site (for example, at the level of director or supervisor), the manager is "in the mist." In other words, nurses at this higher level of management are not characterized as actual people; rather, they are part of some higher, invisible decision-making system. We adopted the term "in the mist," used by some of our research participants, to describe this value generally. Nurses in our research clearly and immediately identified with this term as symbolic of the gap between nurses and their leaders and of the invisibility of their leaders to staff nurses. This value is illustrated by the following staff nurses' descriptions of their nursing leaders.

> *I don't know one. They are unseen to bedside nurses.*

> *Has one ever been on my unit? They are an invisible force.*

> *Who are they? We never see them. Let's hear from them.*

> *They have different philosophies than we do. Have they ever been real nurses?*

> *They do their best. They are dreamers.*

> *They do not represent nurses' concerns or nurses. They don't know our problems.*

> *They decide something, then ask us our opinion after the fact.*

> *They are invisible. They are in the mist.*

Staff nurses assume that, somewhere out there, someone is making the system work. They don't know who these people are. There is virtually no direct connection until decisions are handed down that must be made to work. Even impractical or inefficient decisions will be implemented because of nurses' deeply held value of caring for the system, a value we previously discussed.

The notion of managers "in the mist" is not peculiar to nursing. In other sectors and other groups, higher-level managers are commonly viewed as being in the mist. We continue to identify this value in our research, even in organizations that have adopted new, empowering management techniques. Can the mist be penetrated, or will it continue to exist as a deeply held value in our North American culture?

PENETRATING THE MIST

Once the values of nursing leaders and staff nurses have been identified, the most immediately useful strategy for connecting the two groups, and thus beginning to penetrate the mist, is to assume two or many truths rather than any values conflict. The challenge is then to identify overlap between the values of leaders and of staff nurses rather than to resolve conflict between the two groups in traditional ways, such as compromise. Leaders and staff nurses will espouse either ideological or pragmatic values, or both. One of the greatest challenges here is assisting people in the ideological values group, who find it difficult to develop strategies for working with people in the pragmatic values group. People who hold ideological values feel much more comfortable searching for one truth, which they then fit into their ideological set. People in the pragmatic values group are very comfortable in situations of multiple truths.

We can illustrate the ideological need to search for one truth, rather than acknowledge multiple truths, from our experience with a nurses' strike in one Canadian province. We knew from our data that two truths existed, but health care management (comprised mostly of the ideological values group) seized and acted on one truth, based on the findings of a traditional poll. In this poll, nurses responded "No," to the questions: "Do you want to strike?" and "Do you want to continue to strike?" These responses were truths, another example of superficial values that can be identified through traditional surveys. The value set of nurses mitigates against strikes. Because, the system is identified with caring, to act against the system is contrary to nurses' values.

However, in this case, another value not captured by the surveys was also true. Nurses saw the strike as their only choice, given government proposals for health care reform—proposals that were being implemented by health care management. Nurses believed that government had no knowledge of care at the immediate worksite, nurses' units. What health care management failed to understand was that nurses will act if their ability to care for their patients is seriously compromised. Nurses believed the cost of not acting would harm their patients more than would strike action. In this case, the truth that nurses did not want to strike was all that management needed to reinforce a belief that nurses would not strike for very long. In fact, the strike lasted a great deal longer than anticipated because of the existence of two truths rather than one. A strategy that could have facilitated the strike's end would have involved identifying overlapping values between management and staff nurses. Here, the values associated with caring for patients would have been the field within which to examine values' overlap, because both the health care systems established by management and the caring practices established by nurses are in place to care for patients and clients. Acknowledgment of multiple truths, and a search for an overlap in values among seemingly disparate values groups, are strategies more appropriate than merely identifying actions to resolve an assumed conflict in values or to resolve the existence of multiple truths.

Currently, we are using the overlap strategy in the development of a recruitment style for schools of nursing. The challenge is to use the core value of caring as the field of overlap and to demonstrate how caring includes decision making and other leadership behaviors desirable in nurses. Initial findings suggest that applicants to nursing do not associate behaviors of effective leaders, such as decision making, with caring. Our goal is to find overlapping values so that the holistic, humanistic perspective and the business model of management can be identified as nonconflicting truths about caring.

Our findings also suggest that nurses themselves do not associate leadership behaviors with nursing, although, unlike applicants to nursing, they do associate caring with effective leadership. For example, nurses in our research attach the following symbols to nurses and nursing: "women, helpful, tired, narrow, caring, weak, supportive, compassionate, committed, empathetic, humanitarian, and healing," to mention a few. The symbols they attach to effective leaders are different. For example, the following symbols frequently are used: "efficient, productive, goal-oriented, intelligent, strong, assertive, competent, organized, responsible, caring and powerful," to cite a few. Note that the value of caring is common to both groups. How then, can the values sets of caring (from the humanistic tradition) and decision making (from the business tradition), as well as other leadership behaviors, be brought together? We propose that the use of a values overlap strategy, focused on the commonly held value of caring while still acknowledging both the ideologic and pragmatic values groups, could accomplish the goal of bringing the two values groups together even though, by definition, remote nursing leaders are invisible, or in the mist, as far as staff nurses are concerned.

CARING CAN PENETRATE AND BRIDGE THE MIST

In the interest of identifying common values and using them as the focus for an overlap strategy to bring staff nurses and their leaders closer together, we searched our data further for symbols attached to nursing leaders.

Nurses' remote leaders were viewed as: "committed to health and budgets; caught in the middle; out of touch with the actual work of nurses; unreasonable; autocratic and tough; ruthless, powerful, in charge, isolated, detached, assertive, and political." We returned to the nursing literature at this point because the current debate on compatibility of caring behaviors with business behaviors is central to our alternative proposal for the use of overlapping values.

We asked: Are the nursing leader symbols, identified by the staff nurses in our research, reflective of the attributes identified in the nursing literature as needed by caring nurse administrators, who must also be business-focused? These attributes include, for example, the ability to: identify change as a constant and value it; be a facilitator, coach, and mentor; focus on relationships; be systems-oriented; take risks; care for oneself and support self-care in others; and expertly manage resources (Porter O'Grady, 1992; Wells, 1993). When we look at the labels attached to nursing leaders by staff nurses and at the labels attached to caring nurse administrators by authors in the nursing literature, we do not see values in common. They seem to be miles apart! However, if we return to our earlier discussion of the values that staff nurses attach to effective leaders generally, we find we can use our values overlap strategy. The attributes of (a) commitment to health and budgets and (b) resource management can be interpreted as common to both groups. These attributes can potentially be used as the overlapping field for discussion of truths for both groups. The challenge will be to promote the attributes of commitment to health and budgets and resource management as symbols of caring. Efforts to that end will be enhanced because caring currently is a general value attached, by staff nurses, to effective leaders.

Note, however, that, although the use of the values overlap strategy and the identification and integration of values can penetrate and bridge the mist between staff nurses and their nurse leaders, the value that higher levels of nurse administrators are invisible, and are part of the mist, will continue. Our data from nurses indicate that the North American hierarchical administrative value perspective still holds, despite our best efforts to change it through systems such as shared governance and total quality management. Thus, nurse managers above the unit management level must understand that they will not easily achieve personal, grassroots recognition for their bridging efforts: they are still, by definition, in the mist.

Another challenge that faces nurse managers at higher administrative levels derives from our earlier discussion of the pragmatic and ideologic values groups. The more distant nurse managers are from the new, pragmatic values that are emerging at the staff nurse work-unit level, the more likely they are to use old ideology as the basis for change in the system. When strategies based on old ideology fall short of their desired outcomes, the usual response of managers is to adjust the system (Buchowicz, 1990; Hassard & Sharifi, 1989). For example, no matter where the problem originates, a problem with the *overall system* is presumed to exist, and managers typically will adjust by implementing a systemwide solution to address the situation rather than exploring a pragmatic solution at the work-unit level. This adjustment response is grounded in the North American hierarchical system where the higher the manager's position in the system, the more shielded the manager is from new values in the work unit.

For the gap to be bridged, we must assume the presence of multiple truths rather than single, systemwide truths. Only then will the caring values held by nurses in the work unit overlap with the caring values of nurse administrators who are asked to manage in the new system of limited resources. The value of caring is deeply held by both groups of nurses. We conclude, however, that, in order for decisions about patient or client care to be both effective and believed to be effective, they must be made within the field of the overlap of values of the two groups. Further, given the strongly held value of the work unit among staff nurses, and because these nurses currently represent both the pragmatic and ideologic values groups, problem-solving strategies at the work-unit level can incorporate pragmatic as well as ideologic solutions. Caring is the commonly held value that can serve as the field of overlap, permitting the creative existence of multiple truths within both the ideological and pragmatic values groups. Nurses at the work-unit level are ready to participate creatively in problem solving toward effective and efficient health care, if a system of opportunity is in place that acknowledges their value of the work unit and their potential for decision making. The acknowledgment of caring as the field for the examination of values overlap can be used by nurse administrators and by nurses at the work-unit level as a bridge to create an evolving, caring, fiscally responsible system.

REFERENCES

Aylward, J. M., & Nuttall, G. A. (1994, March 23–25). *Data essential for decisions in the quality of work life issues.* Paper presented at the First International Conference on Quality of Nursing Work Life, Hamilton, Ontario, Canada.

Ameigh, A., & Billet, H. (1992). Caring: A key to empowerment. *Nursing Administration Quarterly, 16,* 43–46.

Brenner, P., & Marz, M. (1986). The care symposium: Considerations for nursing administrators. *Journal of Nursing Administration, 16,* 25–30.

Brown, C. (1991). Caring in nursing administration: Healing through empowering. In M. Leininger & D. Gaut (Eds.), *Caring: The compassionate healer* (pp. 123–133). New York: National League for Nursing Press.

Buchowicz, B. (1990). Cultural transition and attitude change. *Journal of General Management, 15,* 45–55.

Cronkhite, L. (1992). The role of the hospital nurse administrator in a changing health care environment: A study of values and conflicts. Doctoral dissertation, University of Wisconsin, 1991. *Dissertation Abstracts International, 52,* 5757B.

Davies, L. (1988). Understanding organizational culture: A soft systems perspective. *Systems Practice, 1,* 11–36.

Duffy, J. (1993). Caring behaviors of nurse managers: Relationships to staff nurse satisfaction and retention. In D. Gaut (Ed.), *A global agenda for caring* (pp. 365–378), New York: National League for Nursing Press.

Dunham, J. (1989). The art of humanistic nursing administration: Expanding the horizons. *Nursing Administration Quarterly, 13,* 55–66.

Eilon, S. (1990). Editorial: What makes Sammy run? *Omega, 18,* 339–353.

Feuer, L. (1975). *Ideology and the ideologists.* New York: Harper & Row.

Gordon, S. (1991). Fear of caring: The feminist perspective. *American Journal of Nursing, 2,* 45–48.

Hall, E. (1981). *Beyond culture.* Toronto: Doubleday.

Hassard, J., & Sharifi, S. (1989). Corporate culture and strategic change. *Journal of General Management, 15,* 4–19.

Linstone, H., & Turoff, M. (1975). *The Delphi method: Techniques and applications.* Menlo Park, CA: Addison-Wesley.

Lumby, J., & Duffield, C. (1993). Caring nurse managers: Have they a future in today's health care system? In D. Gaut (Ed.), *A global agenda for caring* (pp. 379–390). New York: National League for Nursing Press.

Miles, R., & Randolph, W. (1980). Influence of organizational learning styles on early development. In J. Kimberly & R. Miles (Eds.), *The organizational life cycle* (pp. 44–82). San Francisco: Jossey-Bass.

Miller, D., & Friesen, P. (1980). Momentum and revolution in organization adaptation. *Academy of Management Journal, 23,* 591–614.

Miller, K. (1987). The human care perspective in nursing administration. *Journal of Nursing Administration, 17,* 10–12.

Mowinski Jennings, B. (1987). Social support: A way to a climate of caring. *Nursing Administration Quarterly, 11,* 63–71.

Muller, L. (1993). Empowerers, empowering, and empowerment: A phenomenological study of women leaders. Doctoral dissertation, The Union Institute, 1992. *Dissertation Abstracts International, 53,* 3805B.

Nuttall, G., Farrell, P., Nuttall, M., & Nuttall, G. (1994). *Newfoundland and Labrador Nurses' Union cultural research project.* St. John's: Newfoundland and Labrador Nurses' Union.

Nuttall, G., & Nuttall, M. (1992). *Manitoba Nurses' Union cultural research project.* Winnipeg: Manitoba Nurses' Union.

Nuttall, G., Nuttall, M., & Farrell, P. (1993). *Nova Scotia Nurses' Union cultural research project*. Halifax: Nova Scotia Nurses' Union.

Nuttall, G., Nuttall, M., & Farrell, P. (1994). *New Brunswick Nurses' Union cultural research project*. Saint John: New Brunswick Nurses' Union.

Nyberg, J. (1989). The element of caring in nursing administration. *Nursing Administration Quarterly, 13*, 9–16.

Nyberg, J. (1993). Teaching caring behaviors to the nurse administrator. *Journal of Nursing Administration, 23*, 11–17.

Porter O'Grady, T. (1992). *Implementing shared governance*. St. Louis: Mosby.

Ray, M. (1987). Health care economics and human caring in nursing: Why the moral conflict must be resolved. *Family and Community Health, 19*, 35–43.

Schein, E. (1984). Coming to a new awareness of organizational culture. *Sloan Management Review, 25*, 3–16.

Schein, E. (1990). Organizational culture. *American Psychologist, 45*, 109–119.

Shrivastava, P., & Mitroff, I. (1982). Frames of reference managers use: A study in applied sociology of knowledge. In R. Lamb (Ed.), *Advances in strategic management* (pp. 161–182). Greenwich, CT: JAI Press.

Trice, H. (1993). *Occupational subcultures in the workplace*. Ithaca, NY: ILR Press.

Wells, A. (1993). Shared governance: A model of caring in practice. In D. Gaut (Ed.), *A global agenda for caring*. New York: National League for Nursing Press.

Wilkins, A., & Ouchi, W. (1983). Efficient cultures: Exploring the relationship between culture and organizational performance. *Administrative Science Quarterly, 28*, 468–481.

8

Values, Vision, and Action: Creating a Care-Focused Nursing Practice Environment

Kathleen L. Valentine
Marilyn K. Stiles
Deborah B. Mangan

Creating a culture that supports and empowers nurses to use a caring theoretic perspective is essential to the stewardship of the nursing discipline in the practice setting (Henry, Arndt, DiVincenti, & Marriner-Tomey, 1989; Stevens, 1985). To create such a culture requires both vision and actions based on the fundamental values and beliefs of caring. Caring is "the essence and central focus of nursing practice" (Leininger, 1984). This study describes the context of caring for a larger investigation that implemented two new nursing care delivery systems specifically designed to preserve the quality of care while containing costs. Describing the context of caring is the first step toward integrating caring values into departmental goals, objectives, and professional accountability in changing care delivery systems (Valentine, 1989, 1992). Managerial nurses, practicing nurses, and patients were asked to describe their beliefs about caring. A research-based process called Concept Mapping (Trochim, 1989) was used to identify similar and dissimilar beliefs among the groups. This chapter discusses the study's theoretical framework, background, methodology, and findings, as well as the process of how nurses put their vision of high-quality, caring nursing care into action to create a care-focused professional practice environment.

THEORETICAL FRAMEWORK

Caring is a multidimensional construct comprised of attributes of the nurse, professional vigilance, and nursing interactions (Ray, 1981; Valentine, 1989). The integrated model of caring (Figure 8–1) depicts the core psychological aspects of caring: affect—what one feels; cognition—what one thinks; and interactions with patients, which are focused on teaching and learning or comfort care.

These core aspects are affected by (a) philosophical beliefs, such as trust, ethics, and spirituality; (b) structural aspects of the environment, such as available resources and technology; and (c) turbulent factors, such as organizational change. In this model, the quality of caring affects interactions with patients, patient and system outcomes, professional satisfaction, and marketability of patient care.

In the larger study, the structural environment of caring was purposefully changed in specific ways. New assistant roles, which change staff mix, were introduced, requiring attention to the role delineation and explicit exploration of the dimensions of professional nursing practice.

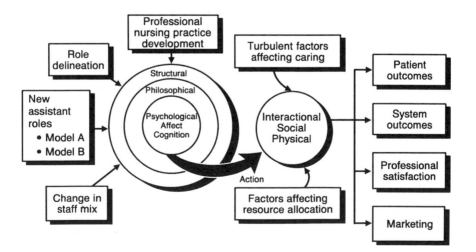

Figure 8–1   Integrated model of caring.

BACKGROUND

A goal of health care reform is greater cost-effectiveness in patient care without compromising quality. The public demands it and hospitals must find ways to provide it. Because nurses are the largest labor force in hospitals, many hospitals are decreasing their costs by drastically reducing their numbers of registered nurses or replacing them altogether with unlicensed personnel whose wages are less but who are unqualified to provide nursing care (Bauerhaus, 1992). Concern that the restructuring of nursing care delivery systems will adversely affect the quality of patient care is triggering a serious and timely professional debate (Bauerhaus, 1992; Berkowitz, 1994; Feldstein, 1988). How hospitals should restructure to balance cost and quality, and how restructuring should be evaluated are not clear (Aiken, 1988; Bauerhaus, 1992; Gardner, 1992). Innovative strategies are critically needed to preserve the role of the registered nurse in the care of patients and to demonstrate, through careful evaluation, that an optimal balance between cost and quality can be achieved (Bauerhaus, 1992; Jones, 1994). When alternative nursing care delivery systems are employed, it is essential that they be critically and comprehensively evaluated. An assessment of caring should be included in the evaluation strategies as an indicator of the success of the care delivery systems.

Mayo Medical Center, Rochester, Minnesota, developed and implemented two new nursing care delivery systems that delegated non-nursing tasks to new assistant roles, changed the mix of registered nurses and assistant personnel, and provided professional practice development to registered nurse personnel. The nursing care delivery systems were designed to: (a) meet Joint Commission on Hospital Accreditation Standards for Nursing Practice, (b) maximize registered nurse involvement in direct patient care, (c) ensure that nursing and non-nursing personnel perform within their clearly delineated roles, (d) enhance continuity of patient care, and (e) optimize patient and staff satisfaction. The models are projected to contain costs by decreasing the numbers of registered nurses and increasing the numbers of assistant personnel. Fewer registered nurses may be needed without adversely affecting the quality of patient care, if sufficient numbers of assistant personnel are employed with 24-hour availability and accountability to registered nurses.

The larger nursing care delivery systems study employs a longitudinal, pretest–posttest, control group design (Campbell & Stanley, 1963) with repeated measures and multiple case studies (Yin, 1989). Eight study units (four experimental, four control) and 1,400 nurse–patient pairs serve as cases. This design permits study of both the short- and long-term effects of the new nursing care delivery systems on the central dependent variables: quality of nursing care, patient and nurse perceptions of caring, patient knowledge of medications and length of stay, and patient and staff satisfaction with nursing care. Statistical analyses include tests for statistical assumptions, assessments of instrument psychometric properties, descriptive statistics, assessment of the comparability of units at baseline, correlational analyses, and multiple logistic regression.

METHODOLOGY

Descriptions of the context of caring were obtained through eliciting caring beliefs of nurses, patients, and nurse managers within the organization, using the Concept Mapping System (Trochim, 1989). This process involves six phases:

1. The group is selected;
2. A focus question is selected;
3. Respondents brainstorm items, then sort and rate these items;
4. Multidimensional scaling and cluster analysis are used to generate concept maps;
5. Participants interpret these maps;
6. Staff use the results in strategic planning.

Subjects

Ninety-eight nurses participated in the Concept Mapping process. Seventy-four were clinical nurses who were chairs or members of specialty practice committees. These committees are part of the governance structure of the nursing department and focus on clinical practice standards. Twenty-four members of the Nursing Management Committee, which coordinates and guides the activities of the nursing department, also participated. Patients (N = 20) and their family members (N = 13) from the "Coronary Club" were invited to participate. The Coronary Club is an information-providing support group for patients who have had a coronary illness, and their families. Patients have had either long-term medical treatment for their illness or a surgical procedure. The club meets monthly and has an ongoing social structure. Members reflect both male and female perspectives about medical and surgical hospital experiences.

The focus question posed to participants was: "When you think about caring between nurses and patients, what comes to mind?" Each group met separately to brainstorm ideas and develop a list of ideas. The brainstormed ideas from the clinical nurses and the nursing management group were consolidated into one data set of 98 items. The patient group generated 75 ideas. The ideas for each group were put on 3 x 5 cards and distributed to them with rating sheets and instructions on how to sort and rate the items. The data were returned to the investigator, and multidimensional scaling and cluster analyses were performed. Concept maps were generated which were then interpreted by each group. Further details on the specifics of this methodology can be found in *Evaluation and Program Planning* (1989), which is dedicated to the Concept Mapping System methodology.

FINDINGS

Nurses

Figure 8–2 is the interpreted map that the clinical nurses generated. Each cluster contains the most closely associated brainstormed ideas.

The proximity of the clusters is indicative of their similarity. For example, cluster 8, "Touching the Inner Being," is more similar to cluster 2, "Therapeutic Relationship," than it is to cluster 5, "Competence." The height of the cluster represents how central the clinical nurses believed the concept is to the idea of caring between nurses and patients. "Advocacy/Cultural Sensitivity" (cluster 1), "Patient/Family-Centered Care Planning" (cluster 7), and "Touching

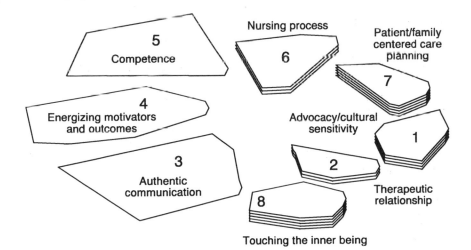

Figure 8–2   Interpreted map for clinical nurses.

the Inner Being" (cluster 8) are central to the clinical nurses' concept of caring, while items that comprise, for example, "Competence" and "Authentic
Communication" are less central. (Details of the items in each of these clusters
are explained in Table 8–1, below.)

Figure 8–3 is the interpreted map from nursing management. These nurses
used the same data set as the clinical nurses, but interpreted the items differently.

Nursing management labeled cluster 1 "Philosophical Beliefs and Actions."
Cluster 7, "Optimizing Patient Involvement," and cluster 8, "Therapeutic Pres-
ence," were the most central clusters for nursing management. Managers also
divided the map into three regions. The region with the most clusters, "The
art of being with and doing," included "Therapeutic Presence," "Creating the
Care Environment," "Philosophical Beliefs and Actions," and "Optimizing
Patient Involvement." Another region, "The art of being with it," included
"Science of Care" and "Competence in Clinical Decision Making." The third

**Table 8–1   Nursing Management Committee/Chairs of Clinical Practice
Committees' Clusters of Brainstormed Items, with Ratings (numbers in
parentheses) for Centrality to the Concept of Caring**

Cluster 1	Cluster 2
Therapeutic Presence/ Touching the Inner Being	Creating the Care Environment/ Therapeutic Relationship
Compassion (4.56)	Attention (3.70)
Comforting (4.29)	Being with (3.63)
Warmth (4.18)	Support (4.08)
Empathy (4.26)	Taking time (3.96)
Listening (4.56)	Developing rapport (4.25)
Sincerity (4.32)	Therapeutic touch (3.81)
Human touch (4.13)	Authentic, letting down pretense,
Acceptance (4.16)	barriers and roles (3.53)
Appropriate humor (3.57)	Helpful (3.60)
Allowing silence (3.70)	Not judging/unconditional (4.11)
Conveying understanding (4.06)	**Cluster Rating Average = 3.85**
Communicating (4.55)	
Openness (3.97)	
Consideration before doing (3.73)	
Sharing feelings (3.27)	
Friendliness (3.71)	
Trust (4.47)	
Cluster Rating Average = 4.09	

region, "Experience of care from the patient's perspective: Engaging in the healing process," included "Interconnectedness" and "Reciprocity of Caring."

Examination of cluster labels across the interpreted maps for nursing management and clinical nurses reveals similarities and differences related to caring (Table 8–1). The centrality rating is on a scale of 1 to 5, with 5 being the highest.

Nursing management's most highly rated cluster (4.21) was labeled "Philosophical Beliefs and Actions"; the same cluster of items was labeled "Advocacy/Cultural Sensitivity" by the clinical nurses (Table 8–1, cluster 8). The clinical and management nurses seem to have labeled the clusters from their lived experience. Nursing management labeled their clusters from a goal perspective, and the clinical nurses labeled their clusters from a practice perspective. For example, "Optimizing Patient Involvement" (Table 8–1, cluster 7) might be a goal or a standard; one achieves it through "Patient/Family-Centered Care Planning." "Creating the Care Environment" (Table 8–1, cluster 2) might be the goal; one achieves it by establishing a "Therapeutic Relationship."

Table 8–1   Continued

Cluster 3	Cluster 4
Interconnectedness/ Authentic Communication	Reciprocity of Caring/ Energizing Motivators and Outcomes
Spiritual (3.56)	Energizing (3.05)
Integrity (4.40)	Exhausting/draining (2.43)
Affirming (3.63)	Ethical (4.45)
Encouraging/coaching (3.97)	Powerful (3.32)
Telling the truth despite the pain (3.70)	Commitment (4.19)
Nonverbal behavior, body language (3.69)	Lifestyle/who you are/your being (3.30)
Intuitive (3.48)	Innovative (3.39)
Painful/difficult (2.46)	Adapting/flexible (3.84)
Altruistic (3.27)	Requires self-awareness, growth-producing (3.80)
Co-identify/interconnectedness (3.06)	Requires personal growth to provide it (3.73)
Ultimate communication: to be understood is very powerful (3.76)	Essential (3.80)
Responsive and deliberate (3.37)	Empowering (3.66)
Involves letting go (3.06)	Rewarding (3.36)
Timeliness (3.46)	Effective (3.76)
Cluster Rating Average = 3.49	Motivating (3.56)
	Cluster Rating Average = 3.58

Table 8-1   Continued

Cluster 5	Cluster 6
Science of Care/Competence	Competence in Clinical Decision Making/ Nursing Process
Theory-based (3.14)	Advocating going beyond the basics (3.87)
Cost-conscious (2.88)	Essence of nursing (3.96)
Requires knowledge (4.12)	Autonomy/promote independence (3.96)
Research-based interventions (3.31)	Involvement/participation (3.90)
Involves risk taking (3.37)	Managing the patients' health process/
Information seeking and providing	potential (3.42)
(3.61)	Assessment/planning/intervention/
Prioritizing/acknowledging limits	evaluation (3.66)
(3.64)	Focus on prevention (3.49)
Collaboration (3.93)	Diagnosing/problem solving (3.53)
Accountability (4.24)	Measuring patients' responses to our
Political/diplomacy/negotiate (2.87)	actions (3.65)
Evolving, changing (3.37)	Professionalism in care (4.19)
Valuable commodity/marketable (2.85)	**Cluster Rating Average = 3.76**
Cluster Rating Average = 3.42	

Items comprising each of the clusters are listed in Table 8–1. For example, in the most central cluster, labeled "Philosophical Beliefs and Actions" by nursing management and "Advocacy/Cultural Sensitivity" by clinical nurses, the cluster included some of the items: "holistic," "humanistic/holistic," "seeing the person versus the disease," "respect for patient rights," "privacy/confidentiality," "therapeutic relationship," and "acknowledgment of the patient's worth." Nursing management labeled cluster 4 "Reciprocity of Caring"; the clinical nurses labeled it "Energizing Motivators and Outcomes." This cluster includes items related to "ethical," "commitment," "adapting/flexible," "requires self-awareness, growth-producing," "requires personal growth to provide it," "empowering," and "effective." Clinical nurses identified that, through reciprocity of caring, they are energized by both intrinsic motivators and patient outcomes. They also emphasized that reciprocity of caring requires openness to growth, which can be empowering.

Patients

Patients brainstormed 75 ideas related to their beliefs about caring between nurses and patients (Figure 8–4).

Table 8–1 Continued

Cluster 7	Cluster 8
Optimizing Patient Involvement/Patient/Family-Centered Care Planning	Philosophical Beliefs and Actions/Advocacy/Cultural Sensitivity
Continuity (3.75)	Holistic (4.39)
Optimized patient control (3.85)	Respect of others' cultures (3.90)
Patient participation in deciding goals (4.23)	Humanistic/holistic (4.19)
A bridge between patient/family, health care providers (3.76)	Family-centered (4.07)
Patient-centered (4.62)	Seeing the person versus the disease (4.41)
Teaching/explaining/preparing (4.21)	Respect for patient rights (4.51)
Individualized (4.44)	Privacy/confidentiality (4.37)
Creating potential for patients' coping and being (3.98)	Being the patient's eyes, ears, and voice (3.79)
Individually defined by culture and person (3.67)	Therapeutic relationship (4.29)
Cluster Rating Average = 4.06	Acknowledgment of the patient's worth (4.45)
	Honoring differences (3.99)
	Cluster Rating Average = 4.21

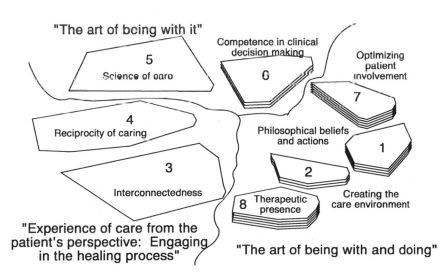

Figure 8–3 Interpreted map for nursing management.

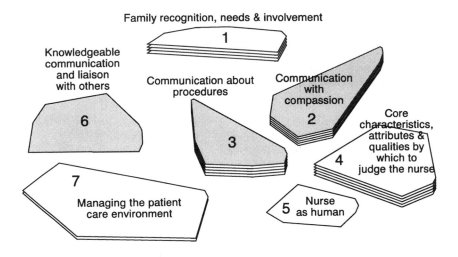

Figure 8–4   Interpreted map for patients.

The clusters most central to patients' and family members' concept of caring are "Communication about Procedures"; "Communication with Compassion"; "Core Characteristics, Attributes, and Qualities by which to Judge the Nurse"; and "Family Recognition, Needs, and Involvement." Horizontally (right to left), the map links communication across the clusters labeled "Communication with Compassion," "Communication about Procedures," and "Knowledgeable Communication and Liaison with Others." The clusters about communication symbolically connect the cluster labeled "Family Recognition, Needs, and Involvement" with the clusters that represent who the nurse is (cluster 4, "Core Characteristics, Attributes, and Qualities by which to Judge the Nurse" and cluster 5, "Nurse as Human") and what the nurse does (cluster 7, "Managing the Patient Care Environment"). Table 8–2 lists items within each cluster.

"Communication about Procedures" (cluster 3) is the most central cluster, with an average cluster rating of 3.98. It is comprised of items such as "help patient communicate when can't talk," "know what other medications the patient is on," "answer call lights," and "on time with medicine." The cluster with the second highest cluster rating (3.92), "Core Characteristics, Attributes, and Qualities by which to Judge the Nurse," is comprised of such items as "be patient," "explain," "see the whole patient," "be observant," "listen," and "hear/understand." As to "Communication with Compassion," patients and families want nurses to "be sensitive to patient/family grief," "tell ahead of time what to expect," "[provide] written information about pills," "[have]

Table 8–2   Coronary Club Patients' Clusters of Brainstormed Ideas, with Ratings (numbers in parentheses) for Centrality to the Concept of Caring

Cluster 1 Family Recognition, Needs, and Involvement	Cluster 2 Communication with Compassion
Recognize family as help, not hindrance (3.64)	Meet spiritual/social emotional/physical needs (3.55)
Recognize family's knowledge of condition (3.85)	Express empathy (3.42)
Leave note to tell family where patient is (3.50)	Be sensitive to patient/family grief (4.06)
Keep family informed of changes in patient status (4.03)	Don't be afraid to laugh/cry/touch patient (3.44)
Keep family informed about procedures (3.88)	Tell ahead of time what to expect (4.09)
Family members present as much as possible (3.52)	Written information about pills (4.06)
Keep family informed (4.06)	Good communication and follow-through (4.12)
Relatives in when patient dying (4.27)	Tell what medicine you're taking (4.18)
When critical, allow family in before procedures (4.18)	Finish procedure before leaving patient (3.67)
Cluster Rating Average = 3.88	Make comfortable (4.03)
	Finish bath before break (3.21)
	Explain procedures (4.18)
	Cluster Rating Average = 3.83

good communication and follow-through," "tell what medicine you're taking," "make comfortable," and "explain procedures."

Families want to be recognized for their expertise and involvement in the patient's care and asked to give information. They also wish to be kept informed about changes in the patient's status and about planned procedures. If a patient becomes critical, family members want to be allowed to see the patient before procedures are done. Patients acknowledge that managing the patient care environment is important, and they want nurses who:

1. Know what to do;
2. Are knowledgeable about nursing;
3. Are qualified to do special duties or procedures;
4. Are always aware of safety;
5. Are rested;

Table 8–2   Continued

Cluster 3	Cluster 4
Communication about Procedures	Core Characteristics, Attributes, and Qualities by which to Judge the Nurse
Help patient communicate when can't talk (4.36)	Be patient (4.06)
Answer questions (3.97)	Just stop by without being called (3.24)
Know what other medications the patient is on (4.30)	Explain (4.39)
Answer call lights (4.36)	Introduce self, give name (3.70)
On time with medicine (4.00)	See the whole patient (3.94)
Back rub (3.21)	Be observant (4.15)
Respect for privacy (3.67)	"Proper" attitude/behavior (3.91)
Cluster Rating Average = 3.98	Listen (4.12)
	Be sensitive (3.73)
	Hear/understand (4.03)
	Smile (3.91)
	Tone of voice (3.85)
	Cluster Rating Average = 3.92

Table 8–2   Continued

Cluster 5	Cluster 6
Nurse as Human	Knowledgeable Communication and Liaison with Others
Nurse acknowledge self as human (3.64)	Adapt to different needs of patient (3.64)
Don't chatter (2.45)	Education about condition before hospitalization (3.76)
Apologize if "screw up," don't be afraid (3.88)	Interpret difficult language (3.06)
Talk TO patient not ABOUT patient (3.67)	Inform about roommate, so less concerned (2.70)
Have sense of humor (3.85)	Respond to concern about roommate (2.82)
Personal appearance (3.88)	Orientation about what to expect from team (3.58)
Present confident manner (3.88)	Acknowledge each patient's individual needs (3.76)
Cluster Rating Average = 3.61	Keep doctor informed of significant changes in condition (4.73)
	Keep non-nurse caregivers informed of special problems (3.82)
	Help interpret communication for team (3.82)
	Know patient as individual (3.42)
	Cluster Rating Average = 3.55

6.   Can gather information about the patient;

7.   Do not come to work with a cold or flu.

Patients also recognize that nurses are human; they wish the nurses to apologize if they "screw up" and not be afraid to acknowledge a mistake. Patients are more confident about their nursing care when nurses attend to their personal appearance, present a confident manner, have a sense of humor, talk *to* them and not *about* them, and acknowledge themselves as human. Communication is important in the role of the nurse as liaison with others—keeping physicians informed of significant changes in a patient's condition, and keeping non-nurse caregivers informed of special problems. Furthermore, helping patients interpret communication from the whole team is essential. Hospital language, comprised of both dialect and jargon, is sometimes difficult for patients to understand, so nurses must interpret its meaning for patients. Moreover, patients wish us to acknowledge their individual needs, and they wish to be educated about what to expect of their condition upon admission to the hospital.

Synthesis

An analysis of clinical nurse, nursing management, and patient concepts of caring revealed that the lived experience of each group is reflected in cluster labels. Nursing management labeled their clusters from a goal perspective. Clinical nurses labeled their clusters from a practice or interaction perspective. Patients labeled their clusters from the perspective of the presence of the nurse in interactions with them. Table 8–3 shows these labels across the groups and in descending order of centrality, based on the ratings. For example, nursing management saw it as important to set standards or goals based on philosophical beliefs and actions that matched these beliefs. The clinical nurses put these beliefs into practice through acting as patient advocates and being culturally sensitive. Patients know this has occurred when they experience knowledgeable communication with the nurse and others. A goal or standard of nursing management is therapeutic presence. Clinical nurses achieve this through touching the patient's inner being. Patients know this has happened when compassion is communicated in interactions. A goal of nursing management is to optimize patient involvement. Clinical nurses achieve this through patient/family-centered care. Patients know this has occurred when family needs and involvement are recognized and supported. A nursing management goal is to create a therapeutic care environment. Clinical nurses achieve this in practice through establishing a therapeutic relationship with patients and families. Patients experience a caring environment when it is managed well. Competence in clinical

Table 8–3   Synthesis of Cluster Labels across Nursing Management Committee, Chairs of Specialty Practice Committees, and Members of the Coronary Club

Nurse Management Committee	Chairs of Speciality Practice Committees	Coronary Club Patients
Philosophical beliefs and actions	Advocacy/cultural sensitivity	Knowledgeable communication and liaison with others
Therapeutic presence	Touching the inner being	Communication with compassion
Optimizing patient involvement	Patient/family-centered	Family recognition needs and involvement
Creating the care environment	Therapeutic relationship	Managing the patient care environment
Competence in clinical decision making	Nursing process	Communication about procedures
Reciprocity of caring	Energizing motivators and patient outcomes	Core characteristic, attributes, and qualities by which to judge the nurse
Interconnectedness	Authentic communication	Nurse as human
Science of care	Competence	(Integrated)

decision making is a nursing management goal that is achieved by clinical nurses through the nursing process or clinical decision making. It is experienced by patients and families when nurses communicate with them about procedures. A goal of nursing management, reciprocity of caring, is experienced by clinical nurses as being energized by motivators and patient outcomes. It is recognized by patients or families as they judge the core characteristics of the nurse. Interconnectedness, another nursing management goal or standard, is achieved in clinical practice through authentic communication. It is known to patients when they see nurses as human and when nurses see themselves as human. Achieving a standard of the science of care, a goal of nursing management, is reflected in clinical practice through competence, and is experienced by patients as integrated within every aspect of a patient–nurse encounter. Patients do not separate competence or the science of care from the affective components of care—all are part of caring. In other words, nurses are only seen as competent if all the dimensions of caring are present.

CONCLUSIONS

Within this organizational context, the synthesis of beliefs about caring—across nursing management, clinical nurses, and patient groups—demonstrated that caring is multidimensional for all three groups. Findings can be summarized by saying: "Caring is visible to patients through the nurse's communication, competence, and coordination of care as these occur within patient and family interactions that are focused on healing." Furthermore, all of the dimensions are interrelated and must be present for caring to be experienced.

UTILIZATION

Study findings have been shared with the participants who generated them. (Each received a copy of the final report.) Results of the larger investigation of the new nursing care delivery systems will be interpreted within the organization's now explicitly defined caring cultural values. Findings are being utilized by Mayo's Department of Nursing Caring Strategic Planning Committee. This committee was established to examine the value of caring within the organization and to assist in ensuring that caring values are infused into policies, procedures, and actions within the department. During a meeting of that committee, members stated that their primary goal was to "make caring visible and explicit within the department" and that this goal could be achieved through optimizing communication and coordination and exhibiting competence in the area of caring.

Communicating this goal will entail meeting with the clinical nurses and nursing management groups to disseminate study findings. Literature on caring will be circulated to provide staff with an opportunity to share their views about caring, determine whether study findings resonate with their own experience, and tell their stories to affirm their values of caring. The committee intends to use research-based results to coordinate its examination of current caring practices and to plan for future practices. The committee also plans to examine existing policies and practices and ensure that the values of care are evident in clinical competencies. Moreover, the committee plans to examine the organization's nursing continuous quality improvement indicators to highlight the aspects of caring that are already present and to develop other indicators that may better reflect values of caring. Departments of nursing in other organizations could use the Concept Mapping System to determine their own context-specific beliefs about caring and compare and contrast them to the findings from this study. Future research could focus on patient satisfaction with the care environment as an indication of the marketability of caring nursing care.

SUMMARY

"Successful strategies are visions, not plans . . . which take on value only as committed people infuse them with energy," wrote Mintzberg (1994). Decision making within the Western health care delivery system has often been based on economic rather than caring values. In this new era of total quality management and patient-focused care, however, a new business paradigm is emerging that is focused on stewardship (Ferguson, 1993; Ray, 1987, 1989; Ray & Riazla, 1993). Essential to the stewardship of nursing into the next century is organizational commitment to promoting visible evidence of the value of caring. As organizations restructure their work environments and consider new nursing care delivery systems that change staff mix and use more assistant personnel, caring values must be included in the evaluation of the success of these strategies. This study reflects one organization's effort to use a research-based strategy to understand the context of caring professional nursing practice. This approach can serve as a model for other organizations as they are challenged to examine their care delivery systems and their values within changing organizational structures.

REFERENCES

Aiken, L. (1988). Assuring the delivery of quality patient care. In *Nursing resources and the delivery of quality patient care.* (NIH Publication No. 89-3008, p. 3010.) Washington, DC: U.S. Government Printing Office.

Bauerhaus, P. I. (1992). Nursing, competition, and quality. In M. Johnson & J. M. McCloskey (Eds.), *Series on nursing administration: Vol. 3. The delivery of quality health care.* St. Louis: Mosby.

Berkowitz, B. (1994). Cost versus quality of health care. In K. Kelly & M. Mass (Eds.), *Series on nursing administration: Vol. 6. Health care rationing.* St. Louis: Mosby.

Campbell, D. T., & Stanley, J. C. (1963). *Experimental and quasi-experimental designs for research.* Boston: Houghton Mifflin.

Evaluation and Program Planning, (1989). *12*(1), 17–24.

Feldstein, P. (1988). *The politics of health legislation: An economic perspective.* Ann Arbor, MI: Health Administration Press Perspectives.

Ferguson, M. (1993). The transformation of values and vocation in the new paradigm in business. In M. Ray & A. Riazla (Eds.), *The new paradigm in business: Emerging strategies for leadership and organizational change.* New York: Putnam.

Gardner, D. L. (1992). Measures of quality. In M. Johnson & J. M. McCloskey (Eds.), *Series on nursing administration: Vol. 3. The delivery of quality health care.* St. Louis: Mosby.

Henry, B., Arndt, C., DiVincenti, M., & Marriner-Tomey, A. (1989). *Dimensions of nursing administration: Theory, research, education, practice.* Boston: Blackwell Scientific Publications.

Jones, K. R. (1994). Restructuring health care services. In K. Kelly & M. Mass (Eds.), *Series on nursing administration: Vol. 6. Health care rationing.* St. Louis: Mosby.

Leininger, M. (1984). Caring: A central focus of nursing and health care services. In M. Leininger (Ed.), *Care: The essence of nursing and health* (pp. 45–59). Thorofare, NJ: Slack.

Mintzberg, H. (1994). The fall and rise of strategy planning. *Harvard Business Review, 72*(1), 107–114.

Ray, M. A. (1981). A study of caring within an institutional culture. *Dissertation Abstracts International, 42*(06), 2310.

Ray, M. (1987). Health care economics and human caring in nursing: Why the moral conflict must be resolved. *Family Community Health, 10*(1), 35–43.

Ray, M. (1989). The theory of bureaucratic caring for nursing practice in the organizational culture. *Nursing Administration Quarterly, 13*(2), 31–42.

Ray, M., & Riazla, A. (Eds.) (1993). *The new paradigm in business: Emerging strategies for leadership and organizational change.* New York: Putnam.

Stevens, B. J. (1985). *The nurse executive* (3rd ed.). Rockville, MD: Aspen Systems Corp.

Trochim, W. K. (1989). An introduction to concept mapping for planning and evaluation. *Evaluation and Program Planning, 12*(1), 1–16.

Valentine, K. L. (1989). Contributions to the theory of care. *Evaluation and Program Planning, 12* (1), 17–24.

Valentine, K. L. (1992). Strategic planning for professional practice. *Journal of Nursing Care Quality, 6*(3), 1–12.

Yin, R. K. (1989). Case study research: Design and methods. *Applied social research methods series:* Vol. 5. Newbury Park, CA: Sage.

9

Patients' Opinions of Mental Health Services in Russia

Andrew Sosnovsky
Kathleen Valentine

Never before has a study been conducted in Russia to specifically elicit psychiatric patients' opinions about the quality of services they received. Until recently, it was considered the exclusive prerogative of Russian health and social policy makers to evaluate the quality of psychiatric services and psychiatric help. This study allowed the voices of psychiatric patients in Russia to be heard. Inclusion of patients in the evaluation of services illuminates aspects of psychiatric hospitals and outpatient establishments that have been previously invisible to doctors, nurses, other health professionals, and families. Information obtained from patients' assessment can play an important role in the development of criteria to measure the quality of services in psychiatric establishments. Caring is present when affect, cognition, and actions are congruent within interactions with patients (Valentine, 1989, 1991). Increased understanding by staff about patients' opinions of quality helps psychiatric staff to create opportunities for authentic caring to occur within their therapeutic interactions.

Historical and cultural factors have, in the past, inhibited the inclusion of patients' opinions in the assessment of quality within Russian psychiatry. A few

The authors gratefully acknowledge the editing and translation assistance provided by Christina Jachman and John Weimholt.

of these factors concern events and beliefs that characterized the rise of communism in the former Soviet Union. Communist ideals included beliefs about the uniformity of citizens' needs in society and endorsed a practice of centralized planning and decision making. These beliefs have had a significant effect on the practice of psychiatry in Russia. A few illustrations are offered below.

HISTORICAL POLICIES AFFECTING PSYCHIATRY

One key factor affecting the practice of psychiatry in Russia is development and administration of psychiatric policies by central governmental planning agencies. The policy makers in these agencies may or may not have been familiar with issues of clinical psychiatry. A consequence of centralized planning and administration is the propensity toward creation of directive rather than participative policies. Such a practice can, in the long run, remove policies from the people most affected by them. A potential consequence is that persons involved in psychiatric care (staff and patients) feel disenfranchised and powerless in determining the nature of their therapeutic interactions.

During the era of communism, there were cultural presumptions about the similarities among people and groups. Sociology, the study of different behaviors in different groups, was not well developed as a discipline. During this era, two practices of psychiatry focused on the isolation of persons with mental illness from the larger society: (a) they were often hospitalized in institutions geographically distant from the center of society, and (b) after discharge, government officials frequently ordered ongoing surveillance of the patients' daily activities.

In the absence of a free market economy, there was little focus on consumer opinion or market research. Thus, the concept of patients as consumers of psychiatric services was foreign to the Soviet citizenry.

The combined effect of these factors contributed to the evolution of a system of services in which deinstitutionalization and treatment of the mentally ill in the least restrictive community setting were not well-developed nor accepted policies. "Psychiatric registration," a form of community practice, was implemented.

Psychiatric registration was (and is) particularly associated with "dispensaries" (psychiatric outpatient clinics). Originally, this practice provided intensive monitoring of patients' progress, after discharge, by qualified professional psychiatrists. Over time, this individually designed intensive case management was transformed into a "rigid, bureaucratic structure that led to social stigmatization (and sometimes even discrimination) of the patients under

a formal and frequently stereotyped psychiatric surveillance. Grounds for psychiatric registration could be any mental disorder, even if it was not severe or
of long duration" (Vartanyan et al., 1993, p. 245).

Although laws were enacted to liberalize psychiatric registration, their implementation has been sporadic and in need of continued reform. For example,
at the end of 1989, 18.6% of all patients who were registered were released from
registration because of the liberalized law. However, dissatisfaction with registration as a concept and practice continues.

Before reforms in psychiatric laws occurred, mounting evidence of a pattern
of increasingly restrictive policies contributed to the expulsion of Soviet Psychiatry from the World Psychiatric Association because of concerns related to
patients' rights. In 1989, Soviet Psychiatry was readmitted to the World Psychiatric Association on a provisional status. The recent reforms toward democracy in the governmental structure of the former Soviet Union are also
becoming evident in the liberalization of laws and clinical practice related to
Russian psychiatric patients' rights.

This chapter provides an example of how Russia can move toward a more de-
mocratic and inclusive approach to the assessment of psychiatric services. In
several ways, the study reported here overcame historical barriers that, in the
past, have impeded such an approach:

1. The study is based on the premise that the formerly voiceless patients
    will be heard and their opinions will be considered in policy debates and
    decisions.

2. The investigators used a combined sociological and clinical psychiatric
    framework. This framework has the advantage of understanding that
    there are a variety of psychiatric settings, and each has different treat-
    ment approaches that may affect differences of opinion observed among
    persons with psychiatric illness. Thus, there is a recognition of the pres-
    ence of unique differences among individuals rather than a presump-
    tion of uniformity.

3. The study recognizes that persons with psychiatric illness have a right
    to have their voices heard. To address this right, researchers used a sam-
    pling method based on recognition that patients with psychiatric illness
    are not always burdened with symptoms that could call into question
    the validity of their responses. There is, instead, health within the ill-
    ness experience of psychiatric patients even during treatment, and, if
    listened to, the patients can help to improve psychiatry.

4. The premise of this study acknowledges that responsible clinicians and
    policy makers seek to understand the opinions of patients, for only
    through collective understanding and action can meaningful reforms
    toward empowered, caring treatment practices be realized.

THE STATEMENT OF THE PROBLEM

Traditionally, the quality of psychiatric services has been evaluated through ex-amination of characteristics, including: duration and frequency of hospitaliza-tion, efficiency of treatment, and degree of restoration of work capability (Averbukh, 1948; Gurovich et al., 1990; Iolovich, & Kopshitser, 1960; Kara-novich, 1946; Sartorius, 1993; Sereiskii, 1939; Zaitsev, Preise, & Ilinykh, 1984; Zelenin, 1948). Such quality indexes became the basis for introducing clini-cal–statistical standards into psychiatric practice. These standards and others established by the World Health Organization (WHO) define the differences between acceptable and unacceptable levels of psychiatric services. Such stan-dards are widely used for accreditation and licensing of psychiatric services (Donabedian, 1981; Leginiski et al., 1989; Seva, 1991). However, such clini-cal–statistical indexes and standards cannot take into account all aspects of psy-chiatric services—in particular, those that concern patients' satisfaction. Even if establishments observed all standards, the quality of help could still be unac-ceptable and lead to patient dissatisfaction. Patients' relationship to psychiatric personnel acquired specific significance after it was proclaimed by the World Health Organization to be a priority principle for ensuring human rights (World Health Organization, 1978). Therefore, research should be directed toward the evaluation of the quality of psychiatric help by investigating patients' satisfac-tion and attitudes toward their treatment (Eisen & Grob, 1979; McClelland, 1992; Sartorius, 1993; Spensley, Edwards, & White, 1980; Weinstein, 1981).

The purpose of this present research was to study the quality of services in psychiatric establishments by evaluating the patients' satisfaction with activi-ties, services, and personnel.

METHODOLOGY

Setting

The research was conducted in psychiatric establishments in Moscow. There are five different types of psychiatric establishments in Russia: (a) inpatient hospitals (N = 3 sites studied), (b) day treatment clinics (N = 2 sites studied), (c) therapeutic industrial rehabilitation sites (workshops) (N = 3 sites stud-ied), (d) psychiatric dispensaries (N = 2 sites studied), and (e) somatic outpa-tient clinics (N = 1 site studied). These five types of agencies provide two general categories of services: outpatient or hospital-based. Outpatient services are available at either somatic polyclinics or dispensaries, each of which has a separate administration. Outpatient clinics offer general health care, including psychiatric services, but usually do not employ psychiatrists. Dispensaries are outpatient psychiatric centers with specialized psychiatric staff.

Hospital-based services have a common administrative structure and are composed of hospital services, day treatment services, and industrial rehabilitation centers (workshops).

Sample

Two hundred seventy-seven patients (109 males and 168 females) participated in this survey. In each type of psychiatric health care facility, 50 to 76 persons were surveyed. More than half of the participating patients had been long-time patients receiving psychiatric services, 58.8% had been observed through dispensary registration, and 61.3% had, at one time, been treated in hospitals. It is reasonable to think that respondents were well informed about the nature of psychiatric services.

In clinical terms, the sample was composed of patients with schizophrenia (8.7%), schizoaffective disorder (24.2%), personality disorders (8.3%), neuroses (17.7%), organic mental disorders (6.7%), and other diagnoses, including mental retardation (35.4%). This sample corresponds with the demographic profile observed in Moscow psychiatric services. Distribution of diagnoses varied only slightly between specific psychiatric sites. The majority of patients in the hospital were treated voluntarily, and five persons were admitted as needing urgent hospitalization. The overwhelming majority of participants interviewed (87%) demonstrated sufficient capacity to understand and answer the researchers' questions and had an understanding of their illness. The exceptions were those with mental retardation, who were sometimes unaware of their condition and needed clarification of questions.

Administration of Questionnaire

Questionnaires were administered, between October 1992 and January 1993, to patients who were treated in the psychiatric hospital, dispensary, day treatment center, outpatient somatic health clinic, or workshops. All questionnaires had a common set of general questions and uniform scale response as well as questions specific to their different settings.

It was necessary to ensure a selection of respondents that (a) preserved a representative sample and the anonymity of answers, and (b) removed the influence of psychotic symptoms as a threat to validity. The main selection criteria were patients' desire to participate in the survey and the absence of severe psychotic symptoms at the time of the interview. The interview responses were conducted anonymously. Only a few patients required clarification of a question, and no responses were dictated by the surveyor. Patients independently answered all questions.

RESULTS AND DISCUSSION

Positive Aspects of Mental Health Services Overall

The majority of those surveyed (76.8%) were satisfied with psychiatric help. However, satisfaction in specific psychiatric establishments was not similar. The somatic polyclinic had the highest satisfaction rating (98%); the day hospital and dispensary had slightly lower ratings (86.4% and 76.4%, respectively). Satisfaction with care in the hospital and workshop appeared considerably less, at 63.6% and 59.6% respectively.

Psychiatric establishments render other kinds of help beyond medical treatment by physicians. Other aspects of care, such as counseling, activities therapy, somatic treatments and so on, contribute to satisfaction and are unique to each type of establishment. Each unique activity was identified specifically for each facility. Satisfaction with each type of activity provided by an establishment was measured. Questions focused on the services that attract patients' attention, and the kinds of services considered most beneficial.

Best Feature of Outpatient Facilities

The comparative analysis of responses to "What is the best feature of the facility?" is shown for the dispensary and polyclinic (Figure 9–1). Note the great variety of responses toward these two facilities. Compared to the dispensary, there is a uniform distribution of positive aspects of activity for the somatic outpatient clinic (polyclinic). Respondents valued the opportunity to have contact with a doctor based on the patient's need rather than having to be referred by another physician (19.5%, and 16.9%, respectively), free treatment (17.1%, 13.9%) and care provided near a patient's own residence (14.3% for both).

Fewer patients positively evaluated the quality of treatment in the somatic polyclinic (16.9%) in comparison with the dispensary (27.1%). This demonstrates not that the quality of treatment is of lesser importance in the polyclinic, but rather that patients found other qualities of the facility to also be factors in their satisfaction. The differences for patients of the dispensary were the

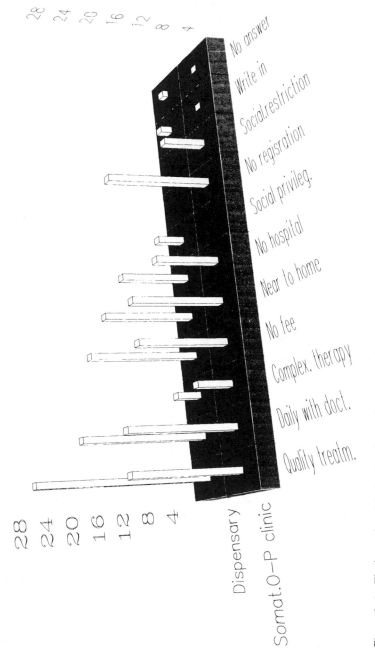

28 24 20 16 12 8 4

No answer
Write in
Social.restriction
No regisration
Social privileg.
No hospital
Near to home
No fee
Complex. therapy
Daily with doct.
Quality treatm.

28 24 20 16 12 8 4

Dispensary
Somat.O–P clinic

Figure 9–1   The best sides of the facility. Respondents were asked to choose only the most important features.

absence of psychiatric registration (seen as important by 16.1% in the outpatient clinic) and social restrictions (seen as important by 6.6% in the outpatient clinic). In addition, the patients positively rated the absence of isolation (10.6% in dispensary and 9.9% in the somatic outpatient clinic). Absence of isolation distinguishes the outpatient services from the psychiatric hospital; hospitalization by nature is isolating. Differences in satisfaction found between the polyclinic and the dispensary may be explained because the patients in the dispensary have had experiences with psychiatrists, and patients in the polyclinic have not.

Best Feature of Hospital Services

A comparative evaluation of opinion patterns in hospital services revealed that the day hospital treatment was more attractive for respondents than was the psychiatric hospital. The most positive aspect of the day hospital was "treatment without isolation" (32%), followed by "daily contact with doctor" (14%) and vicinity to patients' own residence (10%).

For patients from the psychiatric hospital, the most important aspects of service were "quality of treatment" (46%) and "daily contact with doctor" (37%). Activity therapy conducted (8%) and free access to help (6%) were also mentioned.

In evaluating the workshop, patients valued material support (24%), opportunity for dialogue with other patients (34%), everyday contact with the doctor (14%), and living in the vicinity of the workshop (8%). Access to materials is important in the workshop: without materials there is no work, only idle time.

Negative Features of Mental Health Services

Patients were asked to identify both the positive aspects of psychiatric service and their opinions on the negative aspects of the service (Figure 9–2). The main dissatisfactions for the majority of patients in the psychiatric establishments were: overcrowding (62%), mixed diagnoses and severity of patients' illness (52% in hospital, 66% in workshop), bad sanitary conditions (18% in hospital, 30% in workshop), poor quality of meals and insufficient food (24% in day clinic, 34% in workshop), lack of surrounding amenities (8% in day clinic, 24% in hospital), and lack of leisure activities/hobbies (22% in day clinic, 36% in workshop).

Besides these concerns, hospital patients were dissatisfied with the consequences of hospitalization. The most common problems were restriction of work

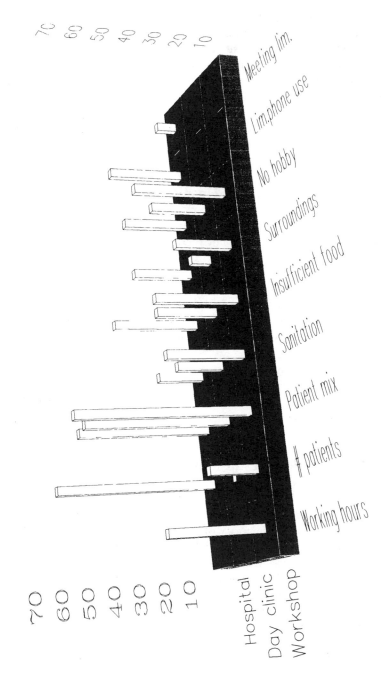

Figure 9-2 Problems with ward conditions (responses only).

(66%), restriction of freedom, connected with the act of hospitalization (48%), and restriction on visitation by parents and relatives (40%). Another protest registered by patients was against the compulsory nature of industrial rehabilitation (36%). About one-third of patients (28%) demanded the elimination of compulsory labor therapies in the psychiatric hospital. As patients begin to recover, they recognize the menial nature of the work, and performing menial tasks leaves them feeling demoralized.

For the dispensary, the patients' most significant concerns were: the availability of medical information to nonmedical establishment officials (58.1%), absence of legal help and support (50%), and restrictions on receiving any information about their own condition or diagnosis (39.3%). The compulsory nature of psychiatric observation and the registration in the dispensary were concerns for 32.8% of the people surveyed.

Nearly one half of the respondents in the dispensary (47.4%) had been confronted with various kinds of restrictions: social 13.2%, and labor 14.5%. Patients thought that these social and professional work limitations were not needed and that this practice represents a very serious problem with the mission of psychiatric establishments.

Respondents' satisfaction with the quality of successful treatment was connected with administration of medications. An absence of medications accounts for the majority (64%) of concerned patients. This problem is especially an issue for outpatients in the outpatient establishments (91.7% in somatic outpatient clinic, 86.7% in dispensary). In activity workshops, in addition to the mentioned problems, the causes for the greatest displeasure were: the limited choice of the work available (33.3%), the monotony of labor tasks (12.8%), and the lack of professional training or preparation for a new profession (7.7%). The day treatment hospital patients worried about the absence of expert specialists (sexopathologist, psychologist, suicidologist, and so on) (16.7%), primitive work therapy (17%), and absence of access to anonymous help (14.6%).

Relationships among Staff and Patients

A separate block of questions addressed the attitudes of patients toward the relationships between patients and medical staff. From the total respondent group, 28.5% of the patients identified at least one form of dissatisfaction with staff behavior. In the hospital, day clinic, or workshop, 38% of patients experienced poor staff behavior, and in the dispensary, the same response came from 27.7%. In the regional somatic polyclinic, such cases were practically missing, totaling only 2%. (Patients could choose more than one problem about which they had concerns.)

The attitudes toward staff varied according to the particular type of establishment (Figure 9–3). For example, rudeness of staff in the hospital and workshop appeared to be two to three times more frequent than in the day clinic or dispensary. It was absent in the somatic polyclinic. Patients in the workshop or dispensary, on the average, experienced humiliation two to three times more often than those in the hospital or day clinic. Experiences of humiliation by patients were absent in the somatic polyclinic responses.

In general, the more restrictive the environment and the closer the staff supervision, the more negatively patients perceived staff; for example, there was greater incidence of staff rudeness and humiliation. In the outpatient establishments, a negative attitude of staff appeared to be experienced by patients less frequently, or, if present, it was displayed in less severe form.

Reasons for Dissatisfaction

The respondents answered a question about reasons for the numerous and serious problems with psychiatric services. In responses from all participants, 64.3% indicated that economic reasons were the most important causes for problems in psychiatric services. All other problems in psychiatry apparently spring from this main source. It is important to note that only 5.8% of respondents considered the problems with psychiatry to be caused by the absence of effective civil laws to protect their valid rights. "Indifference to the needs of psychiatric patients" was cited as a problem by only 9.4% of the total respondents. This may reflect patients' lack of information about their rights, given that the legal statutes have been recently revised. In addition, Russia does not have a well-developed consumer alliance that advocates for the rights of the mentally ill.

Suggestions for Improvement of Services

This block of questions examined patients' opinions on how to overcome the problems faced by the practice of psychiatry. A heavy majority of respondents (90.6%) reported that it is first necessary to improve medical and technical support for psychiatric establishments; 85.2% of respondents believed it would be useful to increase the wages of the staff; and 43.3% said it was necessary to increase the qualifications of doctors, especially those who work in the dispensary, day clinic, or workshop.

Patients suggested ways to improve the attitude and relationship of medical staff toward patients: reward, with bonus pay, those staff who provide the best medical work (87.7%); set up selective hiring based on standards and criteria

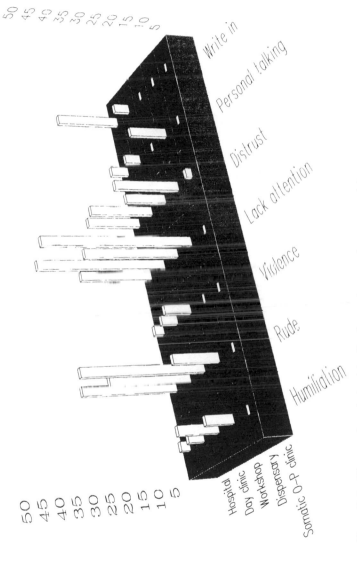

Figure 9-3 The negative relationship, distribution by group (responses only).

127

(66.4%); and enforce serious measures for staff whose attitudes toward patients infringe on patient rights (35.4%).

The majority of patients expressed concern about prevention of social discrimination and maintenance of confidentiality. Patients thought that restrictive treatment environments should be imposed only if the patient is very ill at that moment (72%). Out-of-date prohibitive rules should be eliminated (58%) and psychiatric care should enter the era of "opened doors" (28%). Although, in the last decade, domestic psychiatry has written much about the need for "open door policy," this policy remains insufficiently realized in practice.

Relative to dispensary supervision (registration), from the patients' point of view, it is first necessary to follow the laws that are intended to protect confidentiality and prevent others' access to information about the patient (59.2%). Statutes on confidentiality and protection of information (53.9%) must be strengthened. Patients should be able to demand that registration be removed upon their own request (44.7%) or that registration be canceled all together (9.2%).

Patients want fewer psychiatric restrictions. They know and agree that some limitations are required under certain circumstances. More than half (51.3%) were firmly convinced that the restrictions are necessary for psychiatric patients who present a danger to society. Only 3 respondents (of 76) in the dispensary group thought that social restrictions should be eliminated for all categories of psychiatric conditions.

CONCLUSION

This study illuminates aspects of psychiatric establishments that are important to patients and were formerly invisible to staff and other health care workers. These include the patients' keen assessment of the treatment environment and their desire for adequate medications, qualified staff, and freedom to choose their treatment. Patients were particularly concerned with violation of legal rights and the ethics connected with preservation of confidentiality and unreasonable social restrictions.

The creation of a new method of learning about psychiatric establishments, through clinical-sociological psychiatry, helps to ensure that the concerns of patients are fully explored and reported. With this method, the most and the least attractive aspects of psychiatric services are well revealed, as are the characteristics of psychiatric work that cause the greatest dissatisfaction for patients. Hence, the most important concerns of the public consciousness can be understood. Analysis of the results must contain illustrations of specific aspects of services and be brought to the attention of policy makers and organizations for consideration in their policy deliberations. Policy makers can learn from patients' viewpoints; for example, policy makers have long disputed the practice of placing patients with both severe and mild psychiatric disorders in one department. This study reveals that the patients have a resounding answer to this dispute. Do not mix patients of varying severity in one department!

This is just one example of how the data may be used for improvement of psychiatric services. The clinical-sociological method allows the investigator to more fully illustrate the specific concerns of patients. It is therefore a useful and appropriate method in the complex evaluation of the quality of psychiatric establishments. The planning and creation of treatment environments based on human care theory necessitate the inclusion of a patients' opinions about their needs and experiences. This landmark investigation allows for the voices of patients who use psychiatric services in Russia to be heard, and demonstrates that quality services cannot accurately be defined by policy makers alone.

REFERENCES

Averbukh, F. S. (1948). Organizational-methodological questions about modern neuropsychiatry. *Works of the Scientific Research Institute of Psychoneurology*, 6, 103–113.

Donabedian, A. (1981). Criteria, norms, and standards of quality: What do they mean? *American Journal of Public Health*, 71, 409–412.

Eisen, S. V., & Grob, M. C. (1979). *Hospital and Community Psychiatry*, 30, 344–347.

Gurovich, I. Y., et al (1990). *The main features of activity of psychiatric institutions and the methods of their accounting.* Methodological Recommendations of the Ministry of Health RSFSR (Russian Soviet Federal Socialist Republic). Moscow: Ministry of Health.

Iolovich, I. S., & Kopshitez, I. Z. (1960). *Scientific analysis of medical activities of psychoneurological hospitals and clinics.* State Scientific Research Institute of Psychiatry. Moscow: Ministry of Health.

Karanovich, G. G. (1946). *Journal of Neuropathology and Psychiatry*, 15, 9–13.

Leginski, W. A., et al. (1989). *Data standards for mental health decision support systems.* Washington, DC: 218.

McClelland, R. (1992). *Psychiatric Bulletin*, 16, 411–413.

Sartorius, N. (1993). Treatment of mental disorders: A review of effectiveness. In J. M. Bertolotte (Ed.), (pp. 443–461). London:

Sereiskii, M. Y. (1939). *Collection of scientific works of the Gannushkina Institute*, 4, 9–25.

Seva, A. (1991). *European handbook of psychiatry and mental health, 1*, 317–342.

Spensley, J., Edwards, D. W., & White, E. (1980). Patient satisfaction and involuntary treatment. *American Journal of Orthopsychiatry, 50*(4), 725–727.

Valentine, K. L. (1989). Caring is more than kindness: Modeling its complexities. *Journal of Nursing Administration, 19*(11), 28–34.

Valentine, K. L. (1991). A comprehensive assessment of caring and its relationship to health outcomes. *Journal of Nursing Care Quality 5*(2), 59–68.

Vartanyan, M. E., Yastrebov, V. S., Rotstein, V. G., Solokhina, T. A., Liberman, Y. I., & Shevchenko, L. S. (1993). Russia and the Commonwealth of Independent States. *International handbook on mental health policy.* Westport, CT: Greenwood Press.

Weinstein, R. M. (1981). *Social Science and Medicine, 15*, 310–314.

World Health Organization. (1978, September 6–12). *Primary health care.* Report of the International Conference on Primary Health Care, Alma-Ata, USSR. Geneva: WHO.

Zaitsev, D. A., Preise, X. X., & Ilinykh, Y. A. (1984). Accountings and analysis of manifestations of activity of psychiatric institutions. *Methodical Recommendations of the Ministry of Health.*

Zelenin, N. V. (1948). Organizational-methodological questions about modern neuropsychiatry. *Works of the Scientific Research Institute of Psychoneurology. Collection of articles, 6*, 118–125.

10

Development of an Instrument to Assess Perceptions of Nurse Caring Behaviors Toward Family Members

Lucie Gagnon
Sister Barbara Anne Gooding

The concept of caring has long been central to the identity of the nursing profession. In critical care settings, technical abilities are essential to providing the best possible nursing care to clients. In addition, other strong caring elements are necessary to deliver quality care. For example, caring actions and attitudes on the part of the nurse are important for the client as well as for family members (Breu & Dracup, 1978; Hampe, 1975; Molter, 1979; O'Norris & Grove, 1986; Ray, 1987; Warren, 1994).

A life-threatening illness represents one of the most intense emotional experiences for persons afflicted with the illness and for their families. Often, family members serve as the primary source of support for the critically ill (Chavez & Faber, 1987; Simpson, 1991). However, when experiencing high levels of stress and uncertainty, family members may become too vulnerable to support the ill member efficaciously (Artinian, 1991; Chavez & Faber, 1987; Jacono, Hicks, Antonioni, O'Brien, & Rasi, 1990). In these situations, families have been known to affect negatively the emotional and physical condition of the ill member (Speelding, 1980). By demonstrating a caring and comprehensive attitude to family members, a nurse can play an important role in helping family members deal with the acute event and support the ill member (Caine, 1991; Millar, 1989).

The literature reveals that caring is widely accepted as an essential component of nursing, yet little is known about the behaviors that convey caring, especially within the nurse–family relationship. Knowledge of important caring behaviors, such as those involved in caring for families in crisis, are essential to effective nursing practice (Caine, 1991). The purpose of this study was to develop an instrument to assess the perceptions of nurse caring behaviors toward family members.

First, a research instrument using the Q-methodology was designed and tested to assess family members' and nurses' perceptions of important nurse caring behaviors toward family members in critical care. This new instrument was named the "Family Care-Q Instrument" (FCQI). Second, nurses' and family members' perceptions were assessed during a pilot study conducted with 38 nurses and 20 family members in critical care. Part of the results of this pilot study led to revisions in the structure of the instrument: the number of items, and the instrument's subcategories. This chapter focuses on the details of the instrument development and testing procedures.

LITERATURE REVIEW

Within the helping professions, the importance of caring has been emphasized by numerous authors. As a manifestation of being human, caring is the actualization of the capacity to care, a response to others in specific and concrete acts (Roach, 1987). Behavioral scientists have identified several caring-related elements within a therapist as essential to establishing a therapeutic relationship. These include a desire to help, a genuine liking for others, honesty, trust, respect, understanding of the other, and empathy. They have been stressed as crucial elements that need to be communicated to clients through supportive behaviors (Benjamin, 1981; Rogers, 1962).

In nursing, Watson (1985b) proposed a psychosocial approach to caring, where caring is defined as both an art and a science for nursing. The value of caring becomes a starting point. It manifests itself in concrete acts that are central to the delivery of quality care (Watson, 1985b). Watson's theory identifies ten carative factors that constitute the primary elements for effective nursing practice (Watson et al., 1979):

1. Formation of humanistic–altruistic system of values;
2. Instillation of faith and hope;

3. Cultivation of and sensitivity to self and others;

4. Development of helping–trusting relationship;

5. Promotion and acceptance of the expression of positive and negative feelings;

6. Systematic use of the scientific problem-solving method for decision making;

7. Promotion of interpersonal teaching/learning;

8. Provision for a supportive, protective, or corrective mental, physical, sociocultural, and spiritual environment;

9. Assistance with the gratification of needs;

10. Allowance for existential–phenomenological forces.

Behaviors based on these curative factors integrate scientific and humanistic values and thus are characterized as caring behaviors. They have been further classified as instrumental and expressive. Expressive behaviors promote affective coping through emotional support; instrumental behaviors impart cognitive information through teaching/learning activities (Watson, 1985a). Both kinds of nurse caring behaviors are necessary and appropriate for different persons at different times.

In this study, the notion of caring was based on Watson's philosophy and was seen as an important element of the nurse–family therapeutic relationship in critical care. Caring behaviors are defined as acts answering the needs of family members or improving their condition.

Nurse Caring Behaviors

Several studies have focused on the behavioral aspects of care as descriptors of caring. Most of the empirical studies on caring behaviors have investigated patients' and nurses' perceptions of important nurse caring behaviors within the field of oncology (Brown, 1981; Ford, 1981; Larson, 1981, 1984, 1987; Mayer, 1987; Sloan, 1986).

The Q methodology is well accepted in exploratory research to assess nurses', clients', and family members' perceptions of important nurse caring behaviors (Cronin & Harrison, 1988; Freihofer & Felton, 1976; Irwin & Meier, 1973; Larson, 1981, 1984, 1987; Mayer, 1987; Rosenthal, 1992; Skorupka & Bohnet, 1982; Sloan, 1986). The technique invites the participant to sort a set of statements or items along a continuum of significance (Dennis, 1986). Because the method focuses on the individual's perspective, there are no right or wrong answers.

The Care-Q Caring Assessment Instrument developed by Larson in 1981 has been used in several studies to identify nurses' and clients' perceptions of important nurse caring behaviors (Gooding, Sloan, & Gagnon, 1993; Keane, Chastain, & Rudisill, 1987; Larson, 1987; Mangold, 1991; Mayer, 1987; Rosenthal, 1992; Sloan, 1986). This instrument used Q methodology and comprised 50 behavioral items, each describing a nurse caring behavior within the nurse–patient relationship.

Family members' perceptions of important nurse caring behaviors were addressed in three studies; a different set of items was used in each study. Skorupka and Bohnet (1982) identified behaviors of the nurse acting as a resource person to the family members. Freihofer and Felton (1976) and Irwin and Meier (1973) examined behaviors of the nurse as primary caregiver to hospitalized patients. Behavioral items were developed based on the literature (Freihofer and Felton, 1976; Skorupka & Bohnet, 1982) and on interviews with hospital personnel such as pastoral services, physicians, and nurses (Irwin & Meier, 1973). Only one of these studies (Freihofer & Felton, 1976) used a theoretical framework as a guide in the development of the instrument's items. These instruments make an important contribution to the assessment of caring behaviors, but there are major limitations in their use with family members. Emphasis was placed on patients' physical and emotional needs rather than pertaining primarily to family members' needs. In addition, the behaviors were formulated as imperative statements emphasizing the nurse's actions rather than the affective component of the relationship. Furthermore, evaluation of the psychometric properties of these instruments was limited to content validity. Only one study (Skorupka & Bohnet, 1982) assessed reliability with a sample of ten family members. No assessments were done regarding the degree of homogeneity of the items among the subcategories of the newly designed instruments. The number of items per category was also not indicated.

These limitations of the instruments used in studies identifying nurse caring behaviors toward family members support the need for an instrument that delineates specific nurse caring behaviors toward family members. With a view toward creating such an instrument, a set of items was developed to identify important nurse caring behaviors toward family members in critical care.

INSTRUMENT DEVELOPMENT

The Family Care-Q Instrument (FCQI) contains 50 items; each describes a caring behavior of a nurse toward a family member in critical care. Many of the nurse caring behaviors identified in the FCQI are examples of nurses' responses to needs of families in the intensive care unit, and thus reflect nursing interventions toward families in crisis. Each behavioral statement was elaborated with respect to Watson's ten carative factors. These nursing behaviors demonstrate willingness and intent to convey caring to family members. The set of behaviors contains all positive statements about the nurse–family relationship, with a focus on the family member as the recipient of care. Each item was formulated based on a review of the literature on caring, on families' needs in the critical care setting, and on the literature on supportive behaviors toward families in crisis. In addition, experience in caring for family members in critical care ensured the identification of realistic and feasible interventions relevant to nursing practice.

Each statement of behavior is formulated in a short and simple sentence using language at the elementary reading level, to facilitate understanding. The singular form of nouns and pronouns was preferred, to favor precision and personalization of the statement to family members. Consequently, the nurse was referred to as a female and the family member as a male. The reason for using this language was explained to subjects prior to the completion of the instrument.

In contrast to Larson's Care-Q Caring Assessment Instrument, the FCQI identifies nurse caring behaviors directed toward family members in the critical care setting. However, major similarities exist between the two instruments. The development of the FCQI items involved adapting each of Larson's 50 statements of nurse caring behaviors to the context of the nurse–family relationship and/or modifying Larson's item in order to describe a nursing intervention toward family members in the critical care setting. This procedure attempted to preserve the conceptual interpretation of caring within a nurse–client relationship. Thus, the formulation of the FCQI items was strongly influenced by items comprised in the Care-Q Caring Assessment Instrument. (Consent was obtained from Dr. Larson to proceed with these changes.)

Three different relationships can be identified between Larson's items and those in the FCQI. The FCQI items are "similar to," "extracted from," or "different from" Larson's items. Twenty-one of the 50 FCQI items were qualified as "similar to" Larson's items because Larson's meaning was kept intact, despite the fact that the context was changed to the nurse–family relationship. For example, the item "Helps the patient establish realistic goals," proposed by Larson, yielded to the following FCQI item: "The nurse helps the family member to establish realistic expectations about the patient's condition."

Finally, 15 of Larson's items served as a basis to formulate 23 FCQI items. The concept of caring illustrated in Larson's item was kept, and several behavioral examples within the nurse–family relationship in the intensive care setting were found. For example, the item "Realizes that the nights are frequently the most difficult for the patient," proposed by Larson, yielded to the following FCQI item: "The nurse offers the family member to sleep in the waiting room."

Despite these similarities, major differences exist between the two instruments. Indeed, 14 items of Larson's instrument were not included in the FCQI because they were not pertinent to critical care nursing and/or to the nurse–family relationship in the intensive care setting. For example, the following item was not selected for the FCQI: "When with one patient, concentrate only on that one patient."

Six additional items were formulated to highlight other important aspects of nursing interventions toward family in the intensive care setting, for example: "The nurse explains to the family member the purpose of the machines surrounding the patient."

Content Validity

Items. The items selected were reviewed by four different panels of experts, to ensure content validity. Panel 1 (three nurses: a nurse researcher, a family liaison nurse, and a critical care nurse) reviewed each item for representativeness of the caring concept in nursing and appropriateness to nursing families in critical care. Several terms identified as not clear or probably confusing for family members were exchanged for simpler words. Words such as "convey" and "explore" were modified to bring additional specificity and precision to item formulation. After revisions were made, these expert nurses agreed on the 50 FCQI items as being representative of family nursing in critical care settings.

The second panel, comprised of five nurses with masters' degrees, was asked to complete a checklist verifying whether each revised item was clearly stated, unique, and representative of a caring behavior in nursing. Items that the experts found repetitive were modified to ensure distinction of each item from the others.

Thereafter, members of two panels reviewed the identified items for clarity in item formulation and general understanding. A convenience sample of five critical care nurses and five laypersons constituted these panels. Words judged to be confusing were exchanged for synonyms. Except for these minor substitutions, the instrument remained unchanged.

Subcategories. Two categories of nurse caring behaviors and their subcategories were developed conceptually, based on Watson's (1979) philosophy and theory of the science of caring and on empirical studies describing the concept of caring (Harris, 1989; Larson, 1981; Sloan, 1986). The two categories were identified as expressive and instrumental nurse caring behaviors. The four subcategories of caring behaviors were: (a) expressive-personal behaviors; (b) expressive-affective behaviors; (c) instrumental-physical behaviors; and (d) instrumental-cognitively oriented behaviors.

Five nurse researchers, experts in the field of caring in Canada or in the United States, were given descriptions of the subcategories and asked to assign the 50 statements to one of the identified four subcategories of caring behaviors. There was limited agreement among members of the panel; in fact, only 7 of the 50 items were placed by all in the same category and subcategory. Four out of five nurses agreed on the same category placement (expressive vs. instrumental) for 39 items. For the subcategories, four out of five members of the panel chose the same subcategory for 20 of the 50 items. Despite the fact that the four subcategories did not appear to be mutually exclusive, each item was placed into one of the four subcategories according to the greatest percentage of agreement as to the choice of the subcategory. Ultimately, 17 items were classified as expressive nurse caring behaviors: 8 items were assigned to "personal behaviors" and 9 to "affective behaviors." Within the category of instrumental nurse caring behaviors, 33 items were selected: 15 items were assigned to the subcategory of "physical behaviors" and 18 to "cognitively oriented behaviors."

Translation

The FCQI was meant to be used by a bilingual community of families, clients, and nurses. Therefore, it was determined that a French version would constitute a useful tool for nursing research assessing French-speaking subjects. A professional editor/translator reviewed consecutively both language versions of the items, to determine the accuracy of the translation. This process brought an important refinement to the elaboration of behavioral statements because the meaning of each word and each statement was reassessed.

Procedure for Sorting Items

The Q-methodology was developed as a means of recording and measuring multiple judgments, preferences, and impressions (Nunnally, 1964; Whiting, 1955). Each of the FCQI's 50 nurse caring behaviors toward family members in critical care was printed on a 4 × 4½-inch plasticized card. Each card was numbered for coding purposes. Study participants were informed during data collection that the numbering was for these purposes only. Verbal and written instructions were given to subjects to sort the 50 behavioral items according to seven ranks of importance. A forced choice was required among the available items.

To help subjects conceptualize and enjoy the task, a 29 × 40-inch white rigid folding board constituted the form of the instrument. Three large squares were printed at the bottom of the board to represent the first part of the sort. Above these three squares, 7 envelopes were labeled and placed on a continuum from "the most important" to "the least important." These envelopes were positioned diagonally: "the most important" envelope was placed at the top left of the board and "the least important" envelope was placed at the bottom right. Envelopes were also colored in various intensities to denote their level of importance (bright red for the most important envelope; white, for the least important one). The number of cards/items to be selected for each pile and for each envelope was printed in black. Figure 10–1 is a representation of the instrument display.

Experience has indicated that the task of sorting cards seems to be more interesting and agreeable to subjects than completing a questionnaire. In addition, social desirability, response set, and missing data are almost nonexistent with this method (Kerlinger, 1973). However, Q methodology has been criticized as being time-consuming and difficult (Polit & Hungler, 1987). Moreover, because the Q-sort's statements are ranked relative to other statements in the sort, interpretation of results should not view lower-ranked items as unimportant or unsupportive, but only as less important or less supportive than higher-ranked statements.

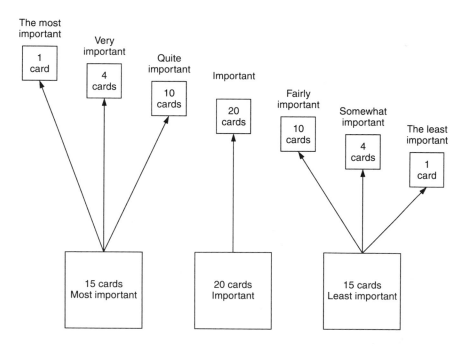

Figure 10–1   A schematic representation of the FCQI display.

INSTRUMENT TESTING AND REVISION

The Family Care-Q Instrument (FCQI) was used during a pilot study conducted with 38 nurses and 20 family members in critical care. One purpose of the pilot study was to test the appropriateness of the methodology and the reliability of the FCQI. Two approaches for estimating reliability were used: internal consistency and test–retest. In addition, reliability of the translation was addressed with a small sample of bilingual nurses.

Assessment of the Sorting Procedure

Responses to the instrument's Q-sort method varied. The majority of family members enjoyed the task of sorting the cards. Many voiced their curiosity and interest when they saw the display of the instrument. Others commented on the behavioral statements identified in the cards and their relative frequency in the intensive care unit chosen for the pilot study. Some nurses commented that the task of sorting the 50 cards in seven ranks of importance was experienced as difficult. The time needed by participants to complete the sort ranged from 35 to 60 minutes.

Several researchers have proposed to investigate familial units rather than individual family members (Gillis, Highley, Roberts, & Martinson, 1989; Hull, 1989). The data were collected from individual family members in this study, but three sessions were conducted with groups of three family members who completed the sorting by reaching a consensus. This experience demonstrated that the instrument may provide an appropriate method for measuring perceptions of familial units.

Reliability

Internal Consistency. The four subcategories were tested for internal consistency using Cronbach alpha coefficient of correlation. Values of Cronbach alpha for each subcategory ranged from −0.33 to 0.08 (Table 10–1). As reported by Volicer (1984), such results may indicate that the identified subcategories were not specific because items were highly correlated with items in other subcategories and were not correlated with one another within the same subcategory.

The items were reassigned intuitively to six new subcategories, which were delineated with respect to the expressive and instrumental categories of nurse

Table 10–1   Coefficients Alpha of the Subcategories Derived by the Panel of Experts

Categories	Subcategories	Number of Items	Standardized Alpha
Expressive	Personal characteristics	8	0.08
	Affective behaviors	9	−0.33
Instrumental	Physical behaviors	15	−0.02
	Cognitively oriented behaviors	18	−0.10

caring behaviors. As mentioned earlier, the category of expressive nurse caring behaviors emphasizes the feelings of the nurses rather than the actions done. This category was divided into three subcategories: (a) "personal behaviors," which refer to the personal and professional attributes of the nurse; (b) "demonstration of affective interest," which consists of caring behaviors demonstrating the nurse's emotional availability and interest in helping the family member; and (c) "emotion-focused caring interventions," which refer to the caring interventions of supporting and comforting.

The category of instrumental nurse caring behaviors emphasizes the actions done rather than the emotions felt. This category was also divided into three subcategories: (a) "facilitation of adaptation to the environment," which refers to nurses' actions performed to facilitate the family members' adaptation to the intensive care unit environment; (b) "demonstration of cognitive interest," which relates to the nurses' actions demonstrating an interest to know more about the family members' experience; and (c) "problem-focused caring

Table 10–2   Coefficients Alpha of the New Subcategories Derived by the Researcher

Categories	Subcategories	Number of Items	Coefficient Alpha
Expressive	Personal behaviors	6	0.63
	Demonstration of affective interest	6	0.59
	Emotion-focused caring interventions	9	0.30
Instrumental	Facilitation of adaptation to the environment	9	0.48
	Demonstration of cognitive interest	6	0.59
	Problem-focused caring interventions	9	0.53

Table 10–3   Reliability Testing of the FCOI: Coefficients of Correlations of the Subcategories

Subcategories	Coefficients of Correlation[1]
Personal behaviors	0.98[2]
Demonstration of affective interest	0.61
Emotion-focused caring interventions	0.99[2]
Facilitation of adaptation to the environment	0.93[2]
Demonstration of cognitive interest	0.89[3]
Problem-focused caring interventions	0.89[3]

[1] Calculated with Pearson's correlations
[2] Significant $p < 0.05$
[3] Significant $p < 0.01$

interventions," which refer to the caring interventions related to the health status of the client. The instrumental nurse caring behaviors include interventions like teaching, informing, and reframing.

During this process, five items were identified as lacking specificity in their formulation and were deleted from the instrument. This resulted in a decrease in the total number of items from 50 to 45. The six new subcategories were tested for internal consistency. These subcategories yielded increased values of Cronbach coefficient alpha, ranging from 0.30 to 0.63 (Table 10–2).

Stability.   Stability of the instrument was addressed in a small test–retest study with a group of six critical care nurses. The retest was completed three weeks after the first completion of the instrument. Values of 0.89 or greater were obtained as coefficients of correlation for five of the six subcategories (Table 10–3).

DISCUSSION

From a historical perspective, the concept of caring has always been central to the identity of the nursing profession. Indeed, nursing has long been acknowledged for its personalized services and comprehensive care. More recently, the profession has focused on taking a family-centered approach rather than one exclusively focused on the individual.

The powerful influence of the family on the hospitalized member's condition and subsequent recovery, as well as the impact of the client's severe illness on the family system, have been reported by several nursing leaders (Gillis et al.,

1989; Wright & Leahey, 1987). Recognition of the family as a unit of concern has prompted nurses to plan and deliver care to families.

Through interviews conducted with critical care families, Warren (1994) reported that nurses who demonstrate caring to a family contribute to providing a supportive environment. The families in Warren's study identified some caring behaviors of critical care nurses (such as informing and inviting families to ask questions, promoting open and honest communication, and so on), which assisted them in coping with high levels of anxiety and which helped them feel more involved in the healing process. Despite all the recent attention given to nurse caring behaviors, no research instrument has been proposed to measure the relative importance of nurse caring behaviors centered on family members' needs in critical care, from the family members' viewpoints. This section reports on the development and testing of such an instrument.

A common problem encountered in the assessment and measurement of the concept of caring is a lack of understanding of behavioral components that constitute caring. Leininger (1988) contended that, to determine a precise definition of caring, the behavioral components of caring need to be clearly defined. In view of the paucity of valid and reliable instruments describing nurse caring behaviors toward family members, the FCQI offers several advantages for nursing research on this subject.

Major similarities exist between the FCQI and Larson's instrument, for example, the structure of the instrument, the content of some behavioral statements, and the methods used. However, major differences exist between the two instruments. Primarily, the FCQI describes nurse caring behaviors toward family members in critical care and thus highlights a specific type of nurse caring relationship in a particular context. Furthermore, the subcategories refer to Watson's theoretical framework and to empirical studies on caring behaviors (Harris, 1989; Sloan, 1986). On the basis of these dissimilarities, the FCQI is considered to be a new instrument.

Considering the relatively unexplored and abstract nature of the concept of caring toward family members, the FCQI provides a foundation for further research studies on this topic. First, the FCQI proposes a unique set of nurse caring behaviors directed essentially toward the family member. The emphasis is put on the nurse–family relationship. The care provided to the patient is considered in the context of caring for family members. Consequently, the behaviors comprising the FCQI conceptualize caring within an interpersonal process, illustrating more than just the recognition of the family members' needs. The instrument addresses also the dynamics of a relationship: its reciprocity, collaboration, and mutual involvement. Therefore, it attempts to operationalize the phenomenon of caring existing in the relationship between nurses and family members in critical care.

Second, the classification of the FCQI behavioral items into subcategories reflects the literature on caring behaviors rather than that on patients' and family members' needs. Furthermore, the testing of the FCQI includes thorough assessments of both validity and reliability.

Third, a French version of the FCQI is available for use with French-speaking families. This may contribute to assessment of cultural differences in perception of important nurse caring behaviors toward family members.

The pilot study indicated that this instrument uses a realistic and appropriate method to assess nurses' and family members' perceptions. Understanding family members' perceptions of important nurse caring behaviors may help nurses be instrumental in changing restrictive critical care policies in ways that allow greater interaction between nurses and families. Further studies using the FCQI are expected to extend the nursing knowledge toward improved care of family members in critical care settings.

REFERENCES

Artinian, N. T. (1991). Strengthening nurse–family relationships in critical care. AACN Clinical Issues in Critical Care Nursing, 8, 269–275.

Benjamin, A. (1981). The helping interview (3rd ed.). Boston: Houghton Mifflin.

Breu, C. S., & Dracup, K. A. (1978). Helping the spouses of critically ill patients. American Journal of Nursing, 78, 50–53.

Brown, L. (1981). Behaviors of nurses perceived by hospitalized clients as indicators of care. Dissertation Abstracts International, 43, 4361B (University Microfilms No. DA8209803).

Caine, R. M. (1991). Incorporating CARE into caring for families in crisis. AACN Clinical Issues in Critical Care Nursing, 2, 236–241.

Chavez, C. W., & Faber, L. (1987). Effect of an education-orientation program on family members who visit their significant other in the intensive care unit. Heart & Lung, 16, 92–99.

Cronin, S. N., & Harrison, B. (1988). Importance of nurse-caring behaviors as perceived by patients after myocardial infarction. Heart & Lung, 17, 374–380.

Dennis, K. E. (1986). Q-methodology: Relevance and application to nursing research. American Nurses Society, 8, 6–17.

Freihofer, P., & Felton, G. (1976). Nursing behaviors in bereavement: An exploratory study. Nursing Research, 25, 332–337.

Ford, M. B. (1981). Nurse professionals and the caring process. Doctoral dissertation, University of Northern California, 1981. Dissertation Abstracts International, 42, 967B–968B.

Gillis, C. L., Highley, B. L., Roberts, B. M., & Martinson, I. M. (1989). *Toward a science of family nursing*. Reading, MA: Addison-Wesley.

Gooding, B., Sloan, M., & Gagnon, L. (1993). Important nurse-caring behaviors: Perceptions of oncology patients and nurses. *The Canadian Journal of Nursing Research, 25*, 65–76.

Harris, J. (1989). *The caring behaviors of nurses as perceived by hospitalized clients*. Unpublished master's thesis, University of Mississippi, Jackson.

Hull, M. M. (1989). Family needs and supportive behaviors during terminal cancer: A review. *Oncology of Nursing Forum, 16*, 787–792.

Irwin, B. L., & Meier, J. R. (1973). Supportive measures for relatives of the fatally ill. *Communicating Nursing Research, 6*, 119–128.

Jacono, J., Hicks, G., Antonioni, C., O'Brien, K., & Rasi, M. (1990). Comparison of perceived needs of family members between registered nurses and family members of critically ill patients in intensive care and neonatal intensive care. *Heart & Lung, 19*, 72–78.

Keane, S. M., Chastain, B., & Rudisill, K. (1987). Caring: Nurse–patient perceptions . . . CARE-Q. *Rehabilitation Nursing, 12*, 182–184.

Kerlinger, F. N. (1973). *Foundations of behavioral research* (2nd ed.). New York: Holt, Rinehart & Winston.

Larson, P. J. (1981). Oncology patients and professional nurses' perceptions of important caring behaviors. Doctoral dissertation, University of California, San Francisco. *Dissertation Abstracts International, 42*, 568B.

Larson, P. J. (1984). Important nurse caring behavior perceived by patients with cancer. *Oncology Nurses' Forum, 11*, 46–50.

Larson, P. J. (1987). Comparison of cancer patients' and professional nurses' perceptions of important nurse-caring behaviors. *Heart & Lung, 16*, 187–192.

Leininger, M. (Ed.). (1988). *Care—The essence of nursing and health*. Detroit: Wayne State University Press.

Mangold, A. M. (1991). Senior nursing students' and professional nurses' perceptions of effective caring behaviors: A comparative study. *Journal of Nursing Education, 30*, 134–139.

Mayer, D. K. (1987). Oncology nurses' versus cancer patients' perceptions of nurse caring behaviors: A replication study. *Oncology Nurses' Forum, 14*, 48–52.

Millar, B. (1989). Critical support in critical care. *Nursing Times, 19*, 31–33.

Molter, N. C. (1979). Needs of relatives of critically ill patients: A descriptive study. *Heart & Lung, 8*, 332–339.

Nunnally, J. (1964). *Educational measurement and evaluation*. New York: McGraw-Hill.

O'Norris, L., & Grove, S. K. (1986). Investigation of selected psychosocial needs of family members of critically ill adults. *Heart & Lung, 15*, 194–199.

Polit, D. F., & Hungler, B. P. (1987). *Nursing research: Principles and methods* (3rd ed.). Philadelphia: Lippincott.

Ray, M. A. (1987). Technological caring: A new model in critical care. *Dimensions of Critical Care Nursing, 6*, 167–173.

Roach, S. (1987). *The human act of caring: A blueprint for the health professions.* Ottawa: Canadian Hospital Association.

Rogers, C. R. (1962). The interpersonal relationship: The core of guidance. *Harvard Educational Review, 32*, 416.

Rosenthal, K. A. (1992). Coronary care patients' and nurses' perceptions of important nurse-caring behaviors. *Heart & Lung, 21*, 536–539.

Simpson, T. (1991). The family as a source of support for the critically ill adult. *AACN Clinical Issues in Critical Care Nursing, 2*, 229–235.

Skorupka, P., & Bohnet, N. (1982). Primary caregivers' perceptions of nursing behaviors that best meet their needs in a home care hospice setting. *Cancer Nursing, 5*, 371–374.

Sloan, M. J. (1986). *The relationship between perceptions of oncology patients and nurses regarding nurse-caring behaviors.* Unpublished master's thesis, McGill University, Montreal, Quebec.

Speelding, E. J. (1980). Social structure and social behavior in an intensive care unit: Patient–family perspectives. *Social Work in Health Care, 6*, 1–23.

Volicer, B. J. (1984). *Multivariate statistics for nursing research.* Orlando, FL: Grune & Stratton.

Warren, N. A. (1994). The phenomena of nurses' caring behaviors as perceived by the critical care family. *Critical Care Nurse Quarterly, 17*, 67–72.

Watson, J. (1979). *Nursing: The philosophy and science of caring.* Boston: Little, Brown.

Watson, J. (1985a). *Nursing: Human science and human care—A theory of nursing.* Norwalk, CT: Appleton-Century-Crofts.

Watson, J. (1985b). *Nursing: The philosophy and science of caring* (rev. ed.). Boulder: Colorado Associated University Press.

Watson, J., Burckhardt, C., Brown, L., Bloch, D., & Hester, N. (1979). A model of caring: An alternative health care model for nursing practice and research. *Clinical and Scientific Sessions.* Kansas City, MO: American Nurses Association.

Whiting, J. F. (1955). Q-sort: A technique for evaluating perceptions of interpersonal relationships. *Nursing Research, 4*, 70–73.

Wright, L. M., & Leahey, M. (1987). *Families and life threatening illness.* Philadelphia, PA: Springhouse Corp.

11

A Nurse Leader's Dilemma: To Care or Not to Care

Sandra S. Sweeney
Barbara A. Thomas

$\mathbf{D}$ilemmas, by definition, require individuals, groups, and/or communities to make choices between two or more equally unsatisfactory alternatives (*Webster*'s, 1951). Nurses and nurse leaders have grown accustomed to the dilemmas confronting them within the context of providing care to patients; however, many nurses remain unfamiliar with the magnitude and consequences of choice making, given the context of the current crises in health care. The nurses' concern and their ability to share their sense of altruism and care for others in special ways are widely known and recognized by many societies, if not always valued. Within recent years, however, the health care issues surrounding access, cost, and quality have resulted in a serious escalation in the number and types of care-related dilemmas nurses in leadership positions must resolve. Aesthetic works often provide guidance and solace in strange but attractive ways. Shakespeare's works, for example, have provided the world with an enduring source of judicious and prudent wisdom. Shakespeare was endowed with a remarkable sense of observation with regard to leadership; a keen sense for discerning human habits, feelings, and behavior; and the ability to ascertain and articulate what differentiates one person from another.

Join us for a brief journey to a theater in your mind. The house lights dim, the curtain rises slowly, and the spotlight focuses on the lonely figure of Hamlet at center stage. The figure moves and delivers soliloquies that envelop the audience in an eerie silence as they behold a human being alone with his thoughts and paralyzed by the knowledge and truth of his predicament. Hamlet is:

- a human being fearful of taking deliberative action;
- a human being ensnared by the unfolding story and drama of a plan;
- a human being tormented by his relationships with the play's other characters;
- a human being caught in an ethical web of right versus wrong, aware of solutions, yet incapable of taking corrective action;
- a human being in need of continuous reassurance;
- a human being immobilized as a consequence of time, circumstances, and emotions;
- a human being who cares deeply and unquestionably about another individual.

Shakespeare's plays and Hamlet's dilemmas are remarkably comparable to the dilemmas confronting today's nurse leaders. Shakespeare's works, the profession of nursing, and the theory and practice of leadership share many commonalities: each is centuries old, each has been the subject of multiple conceptualizations and interpretations; each possesses its own methodologies, its individual cast of characters, and its separate definitions of reality; and each has experienced sporadic triumphs over tragedy.

Hamlet's reality has much in common with the dilemmas contemporary nurse leaders confront on a regular basis. Let us return to the theater in your mind, for scenes from another play.

A chief executive officer (CEO) calls a special meeting of the executive management team and announces a forthcoming 25% across-the-board budget reduction. The nursing department must lay off several professional nurses and replace them with nursing assistants as part of the reduction in costs.

Later in the meeting, the CEO announces that the hospital is beginning final negotiations for a major merger and will undergo, within the year, organizational restructuring from a service-based to a product-line management mission. As the individual representing nursing, you are aware of other product-line-based health care corporations that have virtually eliminated autonomous departments of nursing as one consequence of adopting the product-line model.

The CEO states that full, loyal, and unquestioning support is expected from the executive staff in implementing the pending changes. What nurse leader, upon returning to his or her office to be alone with thoughts of the meeting would not, for a time, be paralyzed by the knowledge and truth of the changing situation? Many might also share with Hamlet:

- a fear of taking deliberative action, particularly in opposition;
- a sense of being trapped by the unfolding story and drama of the situation;
- a sense of being tormented by the ongoing relationships with all of the other characters, particularly professional colleagues;
- a sense of being caught in an ethical web of right versus wrong, aware of what one would like to do and/or perhaps should do, but incapable of initiating those corrective actions;
- a need for reassurance;
- a sense of being immobilized;
- a concern for and caring about the other individuals—clients and colleagues—who are about to be deeply affected.

Nurses, in such situations, often are vulnerable to what I have labeled "Hamlet's Disease." Those with its symptoms become: paralyzed by indecisive, directionless activity or an overwhelming sense of aloneness; neutralized by competing responsibilities to the organization versus the profession; and/or feel compromised because of a fear of engaging in risk-taking behaviors. How often have nurses and nurse leaders found themselves entangled within the drama of the day, living the crises of the workplace at the expense of overlooking the issues of the profession?

Leaders must be able to define reality. Nursing's reality exists within an era of chaos and unreason; uncertainty is the rule rather than the exception; organizational mergers, downsizing, and restructuring define business as usual; and fear and tension pervade many, if not all, levels of health care organizations. Paradoxes are commonplace. The need for courage, action, and a commitment to caring is unparalleled if we are to serve each other and our publics authentically, creatively, honorably, and resolutely.

Who and where are the nurse leaders of today? They are everywhere. They are the nurses who are deeply involved in caring about and doing something to improve the quality of life on this planet, whether for a single person or a complete nation. The nurse leaders of today are those who care about improving the human condition wherever and whenever possible.

We look to nurse leaders who hold positions of national and international prominence—whether by appointment, election, or selection—to provide leadership and action at policy-making levels. Nurses emerge as leaders because of their knowledge and/or reputation for scholarly work, or of their expertise in practice and healing talents, or some accidental circumstance. A few are simply charismatic personages. Most of our nurse leaders, however, remain unknown except to the few who work with them closely on a day-to-day basis. Millions of these leaders direct their power and energy in practicing individualized acts of care(ing), for those actions comprise the essence of nursing (Leininger, 1988).

A review of the literature relevant to the theories of leadership held few surprises. Nursing's dependence on borrowed theories remains very much in evidence. Theories focusing on low/high task versus low/high relationship dimensions, situationally based leadership, or transformational leadership all failed to address the concept of care or caring. Concepts of power, authority, motivation, influence, conflict, control, change, decision making, and affirmative action are abundant, dominant and viable. Perhaps caring is presumed to exist, but its absence, particularly in the nursing leadership literature, gives us reason to pause and reflect on the meaning of its absence. One reference unexpectedly addressed the notion of caring and stated that leaders "motivate personnel by caring for them, challenging them with interested training, developing them into a cohesive team, rewarding successes, and giving them all the responsibility they can handle" (U.S. Army, 1990). Such advice and counsel, especially coming from a field manual of the U.S. Army and not from business or nursing sources, is unusual but typifies the paradoxes that surround the many faces of leadership.

Our quest for a theory of leadership that would address caring in professional nursing ended about two years ago, when we were introduced to Robert W. Terry (1993a, 1993b) and his theory of authentic leadership—the courage to act. Terry's model (Figure 11–1) synthesizes traditional concepts, such as structure, power, mission, and resources, with concepts previously overlooked or given minimal attention by leadership theorists, such as care(ing), spiritual questioning, and moral and ethical manifestations of behavior (Figure 11–2).

Terry's model (1993b) is particularly appropriate to nursing: it builds on the work of previous theorists while adding the dimensions of human action, authenticity, care(ing), and spirituality. The model seems particularly appropriate to power, politics, and public policy. Terry's leadership model (Figure 11–1) revolves around six major organizational concepts—existence, resources, structure, power, mission, and meaning—and represents the relationship these concepts have to individual and to global concerns. When leadership is present, these six concepts work circularly toward achieving authentic action and fulfillment at individual, family, organizational, community, or global levels. The model assumes that each individual is a leader capable of asking essential leadership questions and then acting appropriately. Leadership is defined here as: authentic action; an ethical, honorific, and unique mode of engaging in caring activities that mobilize people to make progress on the *difficult*—not routine—issues they face (Heifetz, 1988; Terry,

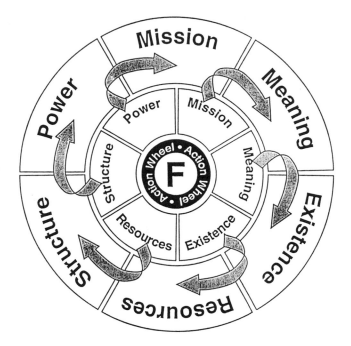

Figure 11–1 Terry's leadership model—an action wheel framework. Used with permission of: The Terry Group, 1900 S. Victoria Rd., Mendota Heights, MN 55118.

1993b). It is our contention that anyone can answer routine questions or problems by following existing policies and procedures. Leaders make progress by solving the difficult noncodified issues of the time.

The essential leadership question, according to Terry (1993b) is: What is really going on? Terry's action wheel framework (Figure 11–1) illustrates a schematic representation of the theory. Visually, the concentric circles communicate its operational messages. A circle is often used as a symbol of eternal life; in this context, we view it as representing the never-ending journey of leadership.

Operationally, one uses the inner circle's concepts to identify and locate the problem; one then refers to the outer circle's concepts to frame the solution. Terry (1993b) argues that solutions (outer circle) are located, in a clockwise movement, to the right of the inner-circle response when this question is applied to a problem: What is really going on? Terry also posits that most attempts to solve problems move in a counterclockwise direction, which further confounds the confusion and frustration experienced by leaders who fail to produce the

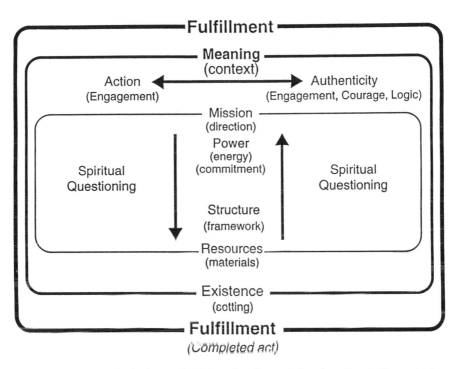

Figure 11–2   Terry's leadership model. Adapted, with permission, from Terry's Human Action Diagnostic Tool.

desired outcomes. For example, if an institution is experiencing restructuring, much of the activity is likely to focus on resources and resource reallocation, and/or one's actual continued existence within the new and emerging structure. The solutions, argues Terry, are to be found in coming to grips with either the power issues and/or change(s) in mission. Thus, the problems and solutions depend on the identification of shared realities—framed and defined, reframed and redefined—until the question "What is really going on?" is answered and the organization determines to rededicate itself to a new reality.

The terms used in Terry's model (1993b) are conceptually and operationally defined as follows:

1. Fulfillment (F)   The completed act *into which* structure, power, mission, meaning, existence, and resources converge at any given time and place. What is the event in its completed action?

2. Meaning — The *why* of action—the specific values, reasons, and rationalizations that justify a particular action. What is at stake?

3. Mission — Any aspect of action that has direction—the *toward which*. Terms such as purpose, expectation, aim, goal, vision, intent, objective, or desire point toward mission; the primary concern for visionary leaders.

4. Power — The actual expenditure of energy; the decision, commitment, passion, and volition that energize a mission. What is the stakeholder's level of commitment?

5. Structure — The *through which* of action—the plans, institutional arrangements, maps, forms, and processes that order and channel power toward accomplishing the mission. What are the plans and processes?

6. Resources — The *with which* of action—anything that is useful, measurable, and necessary for the successful accomplishment of the mission. What are the control and/or peripheral resources?

7. Existence — The *from which* of action—the history, the ecological grounding, and the setting of action. What is the history and/or ecology of this event or situation?

(adapted from Terry, 1993b, pp. 58–60)

How then do the dimensions of caring, human action, authenticity, and spiritual questioning interact with the action wheel? Figure 11–2 reconfigures the action wheel to illustrate how these activities function within Terry's theory of authentic leadership.

LEADERSHIP AND CARE(ING)

Caring is integral to the role of nurse and the profession of nursing. Nightingale (1860) may have been the first nurse to publish a procedure manual for nurses to use in providing care to others, but she was by no means the last theorist to codify this most important human characteristic of nursing. Zderad and Patterson's (1976) work on humanistic nursing, Leininger's (1984) cogent arguments on "caring as the essential component of nursing," and Watson's (1979) text on the philosophy and science of caring have served to draw attention to the need for serious study regarding the very nature of care(ing) in our profession. However, although care and caring have been closely associated with nurse–patient or nurse–family dyads, the need for care and caring of nurses by nurse leaders has not received much attention. If caring is an important integrant for nurses engaged in caring for clients, it is absolutely essential for nurses who are leading others. Paraphrasing Hamlet, our dilemma is: To care or not to care, that indeed *is* the leadership question!

Consider the following hypothesis. If nurses in positions of leadership expect followers to exhibit a caring presence with their clients—whether they are patients, students or colleagues—does it not seem logical that nurse leaders must demonstrate caring attitudes and behaviors with their followers—whether they are staff nurses, faculty members, or other professionals engaged in caring actions? Boykin and Schoenhofer (1993) maintain that "caring is the intentional and authentic presence of the nurse with another who is recognized as a person living, caring, and growing in caring." We maintain that nurse leaders must also engage—consistently, honestly, and with integrity -in intentional and authentic behaviors with their constituents. Once nurse leaders engage in intentionally and authentically being present with their colleagues and their colleagues recognize each of them as human beings who are living, caring, and growing in caring, then perhaps the nursing collective will be able to move forward as a cohesive whole. Nurses perform their duty to clients honorably, passionately, and authentically. Nurse leaders must honor their duty to their colleagues with the same sense of commitment and care. We cannot expect society to value the art and science of caring if we do not value it and live it among ourselves.

The need for caring leaders has never been more critical to nursing. In this era of health care reform, emerging advanced practice roles for nurses, concern for access, cost containment, and the provision of safe care, it is imperative that nurses find ways to provide safe, quality care in spite of the internal and external forces that seem to be assaulting us from every direction. Terry's model (1993b) recognizes the value and need for caring leaders. His work incorporates that of Nouwen (1983), who wrote:

> The word care has its roots in the Gothic Kara which means lament. The basic meaning of care is: to grieve, experience sorrow, to cry out. I am very much struck by this background . . . because we tend to look at caring as an attitude of the strong toward the weak, of the powerful toward the powerless, of the haves toward the have nots. And in fact, we feel quite uncomfortable when invited to enter into another's pain before doing something about it . . . to care means first of all to be present to each other. (pp. 34–36)

Nurse leaders need to rethink and reframe the up–down struggles encountered all too often in their work. They need to create shared experience with their colleagues so that both groups can attend to, care about, and learn from each other, regardless of status, position, and perceived power (Terry, 1993b, p. 185). Depree (1992) describes authenticity in leadership as the blending of one's voice and words with one's touch, that is, one's actions. Terry (1993b) suggests that authentic action embodies that which is true and real—our being true and real with ourselves and our place in the global society. Authentic action occurs when we face our differences openly, embrace our fears, and engage with life toward shared futures. Montgomery and Webster (1993) assert that caring occurs when a nurse develops presence with another, compassionately and respectfully, and allows others to use the gifts of inspiration that enable them to realize their own potentials and maximize their own resources. Benner and Wrubel (1989) argue that caring facilitates the establishment of trust—an environment in which help can be requested as well as given; caring facilitates authentic presence with another human being.

Terry's (1993b) theory of authentic leadership articulates harmoniously with the seminal work in which Roach (1984, 1987) identifies five entities of caring: compassion, competence, confidence, conscience, and commitment. For example, Roach's conscience and Terry's concepts of meaning, authentic action, and spiritual questioning share commonalities related to the moral issues and values that are implicitly associated with a leader's behavior and decisions. Roach defines competence as the knowledge, skills, and attitudes with which one is able to utilize and apply Terry's (1993) concepts of structure, power, mission, meaning, existence, resources, and fulfillment to both difficult and routine issues and problems. Commitment, the human compromise between one's desires and obligations (Roach, 1984, 1987), enjoys a close association with Terry's concept of power—the energy that serves to stir one toward successfully fulfilling a mission. Together, these two frameworks—caring and leadership—can provide useful structures and a syntax for nurses in positions or offices of leadership.

How nurse leaders choose to care or not care is easily determined by their behavior in difficult and routine situations. Leadership is public and interacts in a world of great diversity. Leadership is supposed to work for the common good. Leadership instills hope—realistic hope—and has at its heart a spiritual quest for human fulfillment. Leadership transcends oppression. Nurses and nursing need caring leaders.

We have attempted to share a new theory of leadership proposed by Robert W. Terry (1993a, 1993b) that articulates well with the practice of nursing and with the resurgence of interest in the caring perspective of professional nursing. Nurses must value caring as an essential source of excellence and power in the profession (Leininger, 1984). Nurse leaders must embrace the concept of authentic action with courage, commitment, and determination if we are to assume a leadership role in health care during the next century. We must remain open, and welcome each opportunity to learn and grow. Finally, we suggest:

- Coming together to embrace an authentic caring theory of leadership is only the beginning;
- Keeping ourselves engaged in authentic and caring leadership is progress;
- Genuinely sharing our work, our strengths, our weaknesses, and being present for each other is success.

Let us begin and embrace the caring leadership journey together.

REFERENCES

Benner, P., & Wrubel, J. (1989). The primacy of caring: Stress and coping in health and illness. Menlo Park, CA: Addison-Wesley.

Boykin, A., & Schoenhofer, S. (1993). Nursing as caring: A model for transforming practice. New York: National League for Nursing Press.

DePree, M. (1992). Leadership jazz. New York: Dell.

Heifetz, R. (1988, October). Leadership expert. Inc., pp. 37–48.

Leininger, M. M. (1984). Care: The essence of nursing and health. Thorofare, NY: Slack.

Montgomery, C., & Webster, D. C. (1993). Caring and nursing's metaparadigm: Can they survive the era of managed care? Perspectives in Psychiatric Care, 29(4), 5–12.

Nightingale, F. (1860). Notes on nursing. Connecticut: Appleton.

Nouwen, H. J. M. (1983). Out of solitude. South Bend, IN: Ave Maria Press.

Roach, M. S. (1984). Caring: The human mode of being; implications for nursing. Toronto: University of Toronto.

Roach, M. S. (1987). The human act of caring: A blueprint for the health professions. Ottawa: Canadian Hospital Association.

Terry, R. W. (1993a, April). Leading edge of leadership. Management Advanced Program. Minneapolis: University of Minnesota.

Terry, R. W. (1993b). Authentic leadership: Courage in action. San Francisco: Jossey-Bass.

U.S. Army. (1990). Military leadership (FM 22–100). Washington, DC: Headquarters, Department of the Army.

Watson, J. (1979). Nursing: The philosophy and science of caring. Boston: Little, Brown.

Webster's Dictionary of Synonyms. (1951). Springfield, MA: Merriam.

Zderad, L. T., & Patterson, J. G. (1976). Humanistic nursing. New York: John Wiley & Sons.

Part III

Power, Politics, and Public Policy:
The Education Lens

12

The Curriculum Revolution in Nursing Education: The Caring Perspective and Its Relationship to Power, Politics, and Public Policy

Roxie Thompson Isherwood

Curriculum Revolution . . . As nursing moves into the last decade of the 20th century, nursing educators continue to focus even more critically on the nursing curriculum. To transform the nursing curriculum will mean a transformation in nurses themselves, and thus in nursing. . . . Current models of nursing curriculum development are in dire need of revision or outright rejection. (National League for Nursing, 1988, p. 421)

Such has been the climate in nursing education over the past seven years. Emerging out of the literature for this time frame has been the Curriculum Revolution, a movement by nurse educators to change and revolutionize the dimensions of curriculum development. The Curriculum Revolution has been heralded as a new phase in the evolution of nursing curriculum and, as such, marks a turning point in the development of nursing education.

This chapter explores the Curriculum Revolution in terms of historical dimensions, essential characteristics, and projected features of application. Throughout the discussion, an effort is made to probe the relationships that characterize the Curriculum Revolution, the caring perspective, and the issues of power, politics, and public policy. The Curriculum Revolution can, in this way, be studied in relation to past, present, and future contexts, as well as in terms of its internal integrity. This treatment is intended to encourage both depth and breadth of analysis of this critical period in nursing education.

HISTORICAL CONTEXT

Various authors, using somewhat different dates and labels, have described the developmental phases of curriculum development in nursing education. However, five stages seem to emerge from the combined perspectives of Murdock (1986) and Bevis (1988) to define the field as follows:

1. Pioneering (1873–1893)
2. Standardization (1893–1950)
3. Structural Diversity (1950–1970)
4. Conceptualization and Integration (1970–1986)
5. The Curriculum Revolution (1987–present)

The fifth or current phase, the Curriculum Revolution, constitutes the focus of this chapter, but several factors contribute to a need to briefly examine the preceding four phases in some detail. Writings on the Curriculum Revolution suggest that the fifth stage of curriculum development is as much a function of what it is rejecting as what it is embracing. In these terms, it is critical to appreciate the previous developmental stages that form the bases of rejection. Activity related to the Curriculum Revolution currently centers on dialogue, discussion, hypothesizing, examination, and projection, and gives tentative suggestions regarding implementation. As a result, nursing programs often reflect curriculum development based on previous stages and not on the events related to the Curriculum Revolution. Any analysis of the possible impact of the Curriculum Revolution must consider the nature of current practice as a critical feature in any change process.

Pioneering (1873–1893)

The early 1870s marked the emergence of formal education for nurses. The first American schools of nursing opened in 1873 (Murdock, 1983) and the first Canadian school of nursing, in 1874 (Mussallem, 1965). Prior to this time, nursing care was provided by families, religious orders, and lay groups whose preparation, if any, was a function of apprenticeship training to accumulated lore of nursing practice (Murdock, 1983; Mussallem, 1965). Societal factors contributing to the emergence of formal nursing training included the developing emancipation of women, the growth of hospitals to respond to the demands of population trends, and the need for hospital reform to improve the conditions of health care (Bramadat & Chalmers, 1989; Mussallem, 1965). Into this climate, the first formal schools of nursing emerged as one response to the needs of women, health care, and society.

Within this pioneering period, the picture of curriculum was one of a modified apprenticeship format (Murdock, 1986). Based on job analysis, the curriculum tended to be characterized by mastery of prescribed bedside skills, reliance on ward experience to provide learning opportunities for observation and experience, provision of limited classroom theory at lectures given by physicians, and use of the learning strategies of memorization and recitation (Bramadat & Chalmers, 1989; Murdock, 1986). The inevitable result of this educational system for nurse training was a lack of uniformity in programs of study that demonstrated preference for the service mandate rather than the education directive.

Standardization (1893–1950)

The phase of Standardization in the development of the nursing curriculum was characterized by a drive to create, disseminate, and enforce acceptable standards for the education of nurses. During the decades of this stage, the emphasis on standardization was supported by numerous events both internal and external to the profession of nursing. Internal events affecting the move to standardization included the emergence, in the 1890s, of nursing leaders and professional organizations whose primary focus was nursing education (Bramadat & Chalmers, 1989) and the publication of standard curriculum guides in the United States (Murdock, 1983) and Canada (Bramadat & Chalmers, 1989). In addition to these occurrences within the nursing field, several external events supported standardization in nursing education: the preparation of nursing leaders within the educational mainstream of the college system (Bramadat & Chalmers, 1989), the increased public concerns regarding social welfare and health as a result of periods of war and depression (King, 1970), and the evolution of curriculum as a field of study through the influential work of leaders in education (Murdock, 1983). The climate of the times strongly supported the move toward a minimum standard curriculum for all schools of nursing.

Characteristically, the standard curriculum proposed in both the United States and Canada was based on an activity analysis approach, detailing the functions and qualifications expected of the staff nurse (Murdock, 1986). The intent of the proposed curriculum was to guide schools of nursing in evaluating program quality. During this period, the standard curriculum emerged from the generic notion of the functions of a nurse and served to contribute to significant improvement in schools of nursing (Murdock, 1986).

Structural Diversity (1950–1970)

The postwar years brought economic prosperity, expansion of the health care delivery system, and developments in science and technology that contributed to changes in nursing education (Bramadat & Chalmers, 1989). The expansion of nursing education into college and university settings, coupled with decreasing interest in the standard curriculum and increasing exploration of accreditation, supported a climate that was ready for a new approach to curriculum development (Murdock, 1986). As centralized organizational efforts to standardize the curriculum faded, curriculum development efforts emerged at the grassroots level (Murdock, 1986).

During this phase, school-based curriculum development was characterized by the establishment of school curriculum committees, use of internal and external consultants, and reliance on curriculum-focused in-service education and conferences (Murdock, 1986). Within this context, the need for techniques of curriculum development became pronounced. The Tyler Rationale (Tyler, 1949), emerging from curriculum theory in education, provided the theoretical foundation for grassroots curriculum development during the phase of Structural Diversity (Murdock, 1986). Given the pressure for schools to engage in curriculum development and the lack of a structural approach to do so, it is not surprising that the Tyler Rationale was embraced wholeheartedly by the nursing education community. Factors supporting the ascension of the Tyler-based curriculum included acceptance and promotion by professional organizations, publication of nursing curriculum texts, and reverence for behavioral objectives (Bevis, 1988). Within the context of school-based curriculum development and Tyler-type accreditation expectations, nurse educators replaced standard curriculum guides with curriculum-building textbooks based on the Tyler Rationale (Bevis, 1973; Conley, 1973).

Another major curriculum change of this period focused on organizational patterns of courses. Prior to 1950, content was organized around diseases, body systems, or patient care areas (Murdock, 1986). Structural forms began to expand to include emphasis on student learning needs, nursing problems, and patient totality, with individual schools showing preferences for subject matter, learner, individual and societal problems, or patient (Murdock, 1986).

Conceptualization and Integration (1970–1986)

Within the context of this phase, nursing efforts were directed toward conceptualizing the discipline of nursing, developing the theoretical base for practice, and integrating the nursing curriculum. Several events both internal and external to the field of nursing influenced this approach to curriculum development. Probably the most significant internal event of this time was the growing drive for professionalism in nursing (Bramadat & Chalmers, 1989). This movement provided impetus to the development of conceptual models and frameworks as nurse educators sought to articulate organizing structures that would define and support the nursing curriculum. By the early 1970s, the notion of a conceptual framework within curriculum planning was accepted as a requirement for accreditation (Murdock, 1983). These internal pressures for conceptualization and integration were further supported by the external events of increasing types and numbers of allied health practitioners; changes within the health care delivery system in relation to structures, services, and technology; and the expansion of knowledge within the health field (King, 1974).

Nurse educators, during this phase, sought to define, develop, and publish conceptual frameworks that would serve as integrating vehicles for nursing curriculum (Murdock, 1986). By the 1980s, conceptualization and integration began to be viewed with a more critical eye. Concerns began to emerge in relation to the problems of operationalization (Bramadat & Chalmers, 1989), the focus of integration (Murdock, 1986), and the impact on clinical outcomes (Bramadat & Chalmers, 1986). Although the goals of conceptualization and integration, as with the Tyler Rationale, continued to be evident in contemporary nursing curriculum, the final years of this phase heralded a new willingness to explore alternative pathways to curriculum development (Murdock, 1986). Historical progress and experience in curriculum development, coupled with this receptivity to curriculum innovation, formed the context for the emergence of the Curriculum Revolution.

DESCRIBING THE CURRICULUM REVOLUTION

In 1987, several leaders in nursing education presented papers at the Fourth Conference on Nursing Education, sponsored by the National League for Nursing in the United States (National League for Nursing, 1988). The conference theme, "Curriculum Revolution: Mandate for Change," provided the focus of the papers and the resulting discussion and activity in the area of nursing curriculum. During the intervening years, National League for Nursing publications and nursing education journals have increasingly reflected the growing interest of nurse educators in curriculum change. This movement has been labeled the Curriculum Revolution. In this section, the nature of the Curriculum Revolution will be described in terms of the context for change; caring and the curriculum mandates; and the revolutionary stance.

The Context for Change

The literature suggests three general areas of concern that form the context for curriculum change. For purposes of discussion, these three areas can be considered as the health care dimension, the professional dimension, and the curriculum dimension.

In the past decade, tremendous changes in North American society have significantly impacted health care and nursing. New technology, diminishing resources, expansion of the parameters of health and health care, and societal responses to these events have increasingly challenged nurse educators to consider the adequacy of programs to prepare graduates to function within this context and the context of the future (Tanner, 1990a). In this way, the increasing complexities of health care serve as a catalyst in fostering a climate of critical analysis. The stage is thus set for nurse educators to question the congruence between the demands of professional nursing practice and the skills, abilities, and capacities of the graduate and, inevitably, the nature of the educational experience.

The professional dimension speaks to the issue of approval and accreditation standards within professional organizations. Based on the Tyler Rationale and the trend within nursing to develop conceptual frameworks, many professional organizations have institutionalized the curriculum products of philosophy, conceptual framework, behavioral objectives, and criteria for evaluation (Bevis & Clayton, 1988). The sanctioning of these products has greatly influenced curriculum development as it occurs within nursing programs. Within this context of expected outcomes in the curriculum development process, it is not surprising that nursing education has focused activities within, rather than outside, the sanctioned perspective.

The curriculum dimension, as it is played out in nursing programs, provides a context of unease and dissatisfaction. The entrenchment of curriculum development based on Tyler-type models has resulted in an exclusive approach to nursing curriculum. According to Bevis (1988), the Tyler-type approach is inadequate as the sole basis for nursing curriculum because it supports the technical training aspect of nursing and not the professional education mandate of nursing. The nature of the criticism suggests that a Tyler-type approach may have merit for selected aspects of nursing education, but that its prescriptive, behaviorist, rule-driven features preclude its use as the best or the only view of curriculum development (Bevis, 1988; Bevis & Clayton, 1988; Watson, 1988). Within this perspective, the focus appears to be on expansion of curriculum development views and rejection of single-model approaches.

The combination of societal, professional, and curriculum dimensions provides the contextual climate for the Curriculum Revolution. As these three dimensions interact, issues of power, politics, and public policy emerge, creating dissonance among the multiple realities of health care complexity, professional expectations, and curriculum structures. This contextual background, coupled with a curriculum conference and a community of leading nurse educators, suggests an almost inevitable timeliness for the Curriculum Revolution.

Caring and the Curriculum Mandates

Because the Curriculum Revolution is in an early developmental stage and the relevant literature is based in rhetoric, dialogue, and discussion, it is somewhat difficult to identify essential dimensions without a loss of meaning. However, an attempt has been made to elicit general features characterizing the Curriculum Revolution by consolidating the ideas of major writings in the area. Emerging from the literature is a focus on the caring perspective as the central, unifying directive of curriculum change. The caring perspective is expressed in the Curriculum Revolution through four mandates related to society, education, practice, and relationship. At this point, the caring perspective and the mandates will be discussed in terms of fundamental characteristics that appear to define the area. Issues of power, politics, and public policy will be discussed as they influence and are influenced by the Curriculum Revolution.

The caring perspective, although somewhat difficult to articulate, is the fundamental, essential dimension of the Curriculum Revolution and is expressed through the contexts of the four mandates. Within the literature, authors characterize caring as the central moral value in the practice of nursing (Bevis, 1989; Diekelmann, 1990; Roach, 1991; Tanner, 1990b; Watson, 1988). Although the concept of caring is not unique to nursing, the moral imperative of caring is viewed as unique in nursing in the sense that it is expressed within professional practice (Roach, 1991). Caring is seen as the fundamental value that defines nursing practice in service, education, and research, thus transcending setting and focus (Diekelmann, 1990). Regardless of context, caring is the factor that allows understanding and action related to client issues (Tanner,

1990b). The caring imperative is central to nursing's ability to serve society, clients, nurses, and students, and can be expressed through the philosophies, theories, and beliefs that guide practice and through practice itself.

In relation to the specific circumstances of nursing education, caring is viewed as a victim of the rationalist–objectivist model of education (Watson, 1988). Caring, as the central value in professional practice, defies the requirements of the technical training model and challenges nursing education to attend to congruence between curricular practices and professional care expectations. In this way, nurse educators are asked to reconsider all aspects of nursing curriculum in terms of the caring directive (Watson, 1988), with the view of caring as fundamental to the curriculum (Bevis, 1989).

Several researchers within the nursing community have contributed to the primacy of caring in the Curriculum Revolution (Bevis, 1989). Over the past decade, writing, speaking, and researching in the area of caring have increased considerably and have heightened the importance of grounding all aspects of nursing practice in the concept of caring. The caring perspective has also been influenced by feminist thought, which projects links among women, caring, and power (Watson, 1990). Within this feminist perspective, caring is seen as a potentially powerful tool to transform health care through nursing practice. Caring has thus assumed a central position in the nursing literature, thereby requiring nursing education to reflect on caring in the curriculum.

The literature of the Curriculum Revolution suggests that the caring perspective is expressed in a society mandate that acknowledges the importance of the societal and health care contexts and the related social and political action in nursing education. Within the social context, nursing faces health problems that are primarily a function of environment and lifestyle conditions resulting from socioeconomic/political realities (Donley, 1989; Chopoorian, 1990; Watson, 1990). The health care system, in contrast, remains disease-driven and individual-focused, failing to respond to health conditions that arise out of social, economic, and political inequities (Chopoorian, 1990). Functioning within the traditional health care system, nursing struggles with the discrepancies between societal need and treatment priorities. This imbalance between society's health realities and health care's inadequate responses forms the basis for the society mandate in the Curriculum Revolution.

Grounded in a sense of social responsibility, nurse educators seek to broaden the education experience to include an action stance. Including a social action agenda in curriculum development is viewed as one way that nursing can respond to the need to transform health care (Moccia, 1990). In facilitating this change in orientation, educators need to consider ways of integrating socioeconomic/political consciousness, critique, and action into nursing curriculum (Chopoorian, 1990).

Literature underpinning the society mandate is primarily related to feminist approaches and social action theory (Chopoorian, 1990; Moccia, 1990; Watson, 1990). From these perspectives, the health care system is viewed as a patriarchal structure rooted in practices of control and dominance that significantly interfere with responsiveness to societal needs. The society mandate encourages nurse educators to enable individuals to prepare themselves for the task of challenging the patriarchal values of the health care system (Moccia, 1990). In addition to focusing on preparation of self and of nursing students, a logical extension of this theme would include the enabling of client populations to interact with the health care system in a more meaningful way.

The education mandate, as it gives voice to the caring perspective, is perhaps the most clearly articulated and possibly the most familiar dimension of the Curriculum Revolution. Within this context, the general thrust of the argument is based on the concept of theoretical pluralism as the driving force for new approaches in nursing education (Tanner, 1990a). Nurse educators are encouraged to reject singular and narrow views and embrace the notion of experimentation from multiple theoretical perspectives (Tanner, 1990b). It is anticipated that the commitment to multiple perspectives will challenge, expand, and enhance our vision of what constitutes quality nursing education. Overall, the view is that theoretical pluralism will contribute to a richer mix in nursing curriculum by emphasizing dimensions inherent in professional education, thus moving beyond the restrictions of prescriptive approaches. Implicit in this view is resistance to any one perspective, even a "new" one, and acceptance of a wide variety of approaches in the spirit of diversity and experimentation (Tanner, 1990b).

In addition to proposing theoretical pluralism, the educational mandate challenges us to reconceptualize our understanding of what constitutes legitimate learning experiences and outcomes. The literature uses a variety of terminology in relation to an emphasis on creative and critical thinking as the essential basis for learning activities in nursing education. Although authors may express this change in terms of higher types of learning (Bevis, 1988) or more complex levels of cognitive development (Valiga, 1988), the basic premise appears to be an increasing concern with viewing wholes, developing insights, and interpreting meanings, and using critical inquiry processes (Allen, 1990; Bevis, 1989; Diekelmann, 1990; Valiga, 1988). The literature also suggests that this revisioning of educative intentions necessitates fundamental changes in how educators view content, teacher–student interaction, teacher–student roles, and theory–practice relationships. Because many of these areas are addressed in subsequent sections of this chapter, further discussion is not considered appropriate here. It is perhaps enough to comment that educators are urging that an interpretative stance is in order, so that the fundamental features of teaching and learning and the related means of conceptualization and operationalization are subjected to reflection in terms of congruence with educative, not simply training, perspectives (Tanner, 1990b).

The literature that contributes to the development of the education mandate emerges from multiple sources. Consistent with the historical relationships between the fields of education and nursing, nurse educators have been influenced by events occurring in such areas of study as curriculum development, learning theory, and cognitive psychology (Bevis, 1988). Research conducted within the nursing community is also beginning to impact nurse educators in relation to the practice of nursing education. Over the past decade, nursing philosophy and research have experienced a paradigm shift from a traditional medical-model focus to a more humanistic perspective (Bevis, 1990). The education mandate suggests that nursing education is beginning to address similar issues.

Traditionally, practice has been conceptualized as the application of knowledge in the clinical area (Tanner, 1990b). Consistent with the technical mode of practice, classroom teaching or "theory" is applied to practice in the "clinical" setting. The practice mandate rejects this view of practice, suggesting that professional education requires that theory and practice be envisioned as a codependent pair comprising a whole. Within the caring perspective of the Curriculum Revolution, theory informs practice and practice informs theory, thereby creating a contextual, reality-based forum for learning (Bevis, 1989). This significantly changes the "ugly sister" status of clinical practice, whereby theoretical knowledge reigns supreme and the practice setting constitutes simply a forum for application. Replacing the notion of the dichotomy of theory (classroom knowledge) and practice (application of classroom knowledge), the practice mandate proposes that these concepts be merged in recognition of the complexities of interrelatedness that characterize them (Bevis, 1988). Just as theory is not practice-free, so too practice is not theory-free. Theory and practice assume meaning through, around, and in relation to each other (Bevis, 1988). In nursing education, understanding requires that learning be situated in theory–practice moments that, by their very nature, are relevant, contextual, and real-life (Moccia, 1990; Tanner, 1988). Such experiences challenge any attempts to return to the simplistic theory-to-application approach.

In the past decade, the use of rationalist models to explain clinical abilities in the practice setting has been significantly challenged. Exploratory work in education and nursing in relation to ways of knowing, development of expertise, and role of intuition have contributed to the reevaluation of theory–practice relationships in nursing education (Bevis, 1989; Tanner, 1988).

Few authors fail to address issues related to dialogue, partnership, interaction, or relationship in their writings about the Curriculum Revolution. In the literature, the call for reform of the teacher–student relationship is noteworthy in its universality. The caring perspective as expressed in the relationship mandate speaks clearly for a revisioning of the teacher–student relationship, maintaining that the essence of curriculum rests in the quality of interaction (Bevis, 1989). Within this revisioning, changes in educational intentions, power relationships, and role expectations are considered to be essential to the creation of an egalitarian, cooperative educational community (Moccia, 1990).

In the creation of a new educational community, the intentions of nurse educators center on fostering a sense of agency, a sense of responsibility and accountability, and a sense of connection in both teachers and students (Moccia, 1990). These three fundamental feelings reflect beliefs in the ability of individuals to act with impact, the responsibility of individuals to account for action to themselves and their communities, and the right of individuals to share a sense of community relationship (Moccia, 1990). If these beliefs are to be operationalized in any real sense in nursing education, it is necessary to think of curriculum as the educational community. This sense of community with teachers and students and their transactions as the fundamental, defining feature challenges some of the basic assumptions of the behavioral approach in terms of power, control, autonomy, and role relationships.

The relationship mandate is concerned with power and empowerment as a fundamental concern in the educational community. Rather than addressing power issues in quantitative terms of shifts or sharing, this mandate focuses on power as empowerment of the group and its membership (Chinn, 1989). Power as enacted in teaching and learning can be seen as related to the educational intentions within the community, forming powers of collectivity, unity, sharing, integration, diversity, consciousness, responsibility, intuition, nurturing, and process (Chinn, 1989). Within this context, power is viewed as a function of the whole and is situated in opposition to the authoritarian models of education that seek to control students through rigidly prescribed structures in the curriculum (Allen, 1990).

Within the relationship mandate, the responsibility for learning is shared by teacher and student as it is acted out in interactions within the educational community (Tanner, 1990b). Teacher–student roles that emerge from behaviorist models as based in power position and prescription must be transformed (Bevis, 1988). The notion of equal partnership suggests that teacher–student interaction must be characterized by active, interactive participation (Bevis, 1990), shared decision making (Diekelmann, 1989), and role flexibility (Diekelmann, 1989). Within this framework, the student is considered to be a fully participating member of the community, whose worth, intelligence, dignity, and experiences bring unique features to the learning environment (Bevis, 1988). Teacher and student contribute to an educational community in which dialogue, interaction, and transactions form the basis for learning within the curriculum.

The relationship mandate is based in the concept of liberation for both teachers and students. In moving beyond the behaviorist stance, teachers and students are freed from prescriptions and power relationships that are restrictive to both parties. They are invited to enter a world of dialogue where flexibility, negotiation, and relevance are possible within community perspectives (Allen, 1990).

The Revolutionary Stance

The term *revolution* has been the subject of mixed review. For some nurse educators, the notion of revolution is grounded in chaos and destruction and, as such, is a difficult and threatening term (Bevis, 1989). For others, the concept of revolution is an exciting opportunity that heralds dramatic transformations (Moccia, 1990). Regardless of the value-laden response to the term, there is some evidence that the Curriculum Revolution constitutes a revolution in process. The Curriculum Revolution has been characterized as revolutionary in intent, rather than innovative or reforming (Tanner, 1990b). Supporting this position are the features of alternative conceptions of education, reflection of major social change, and expectation of new ends (Tanner, 1990b). It seems apparent that the Curriculum Revolution is proposing a new worldview of nursing education, including changes in the ways that power, politics, and public policy are constituted in curriculum development. However, it is a revolution in progress; its future impact rests on the development of a new paradigm, the persuasiveness of the change proposed, and the receptivity of the community of nursing education.

Within the literature, several nurse educators have suggested some concerns that may impact the progress of the Curriculum Revolution. One area of concern is the possibility that the revolution may divide, rather than unite, nurse educators along program lines, interest areas, or interpretative conflicts (Bevis, 1989). A second concern relates to replacing one dogma with another in our inability to tolerate the fundamental complexity, flexibility, and ill-structuredness of the Curriculum Revolution (Bevis, 1990; Donley, 1989). If the tenets of the Curriculum Revolution are interpreted as prescriptive entities, rather than guiding principles, then nursing education has substituted one set of rules for another. A third area of concern centers around the issue of destroying the old and embracing the new. Although the Curriculum Revolution may appear to wholeheartedly reject behaviorist models of education, several nurse educators caution against this interpretation, maintaining a commitment to theoretical pluralism that includes consideration of previously held frameworks (Bevis, 1988; deTornyay, 1990). These three cautions are significant considerations in the evolution of the Curriculum Revolution; they provide some indicators of potential problem areas and thus serve to guide both the converted and the yet-to-be-converted in their critique of the progress of the revolutionary movement.

APPLYING THE CURRICULUM REVOLUTION

The writings of the Curriculum Revolution indicate that nurse educators have begun to address the challenges of implementation. It is beyond the confines of this chapter to explore the literature that describes application efforts related to the Curriculum Revolution. However, much of the recent research and scholarly investigation appears to focus on the caring perspective and its relationship to pedagogical issues (Appleton, 1990; Beck, 1992; Diekelmann, 1992, 1993; Halldorsdottir, 1990; Hughes, 1992, 1993; Miller, Haber, & Byrne, 1990). Earlier operationalization efforts usually took the form of discussion papers characterized by attention to a particular feature or mandate, or broad generalizations of possible activities, with few examples of situation-specific approaches. At this point in time, the literature related to the Curriculum Revolution appears to be defined by a number of general thematic areas that are grounded in theoretical perspectives but lack a distinct conceptual framework, modes of implementation, and a track record in research.

It would take a greater thinker than I to project what comprehensive curriculum development would look like within the approaches of the Curriculum Revolution. Most applications are currently conceived as parts of an undeveloped whole. As such, they appear as isolated principles or suggestions, involving promotion of interactive modes of teaching and learning, increased faculty and student involvement in curricular decision making, and greater program autonomy in curriculum development. The preliminary stage of development suggests that it might be appropriate to focus application discussion on strategic points of preparation, these being some of the areas requiring intensive consideration if the tenets of the Curriculum Revolution are going to grow to fruition. Inevitably, these points of preparation are profoundly related to the structures, roles, and functions that influence and are influenced by changes in power, politics, and public polity. These preparation points and some of the possible areas of relevance are contextualized here around the perspectives of student, teacher, faculty/program, institution, community, and professional organization:

Student Preparation

- Progressive development of abilities to engage in curriculum in terms of participation, expectation, and structure.
- Utilization of individual background in terms of experience, interest, and motivation.
- Increasing autonomy as a member of the educational community.
- Reallocation of personal resources in the educational experience.

Teacher Preparation

- Emphasis on development of interactive teaching perspectives.
- Assistance in moving from a Tyler-based stance to a cooperative, interactive stance in relation to curriculum inquiry.
- Encouragement of scholarship in terms of curriculum creations.
- Leadership in pioneering creative applications of the Curriculum Revolution.
- Responsibility in acting as a catalyst in the creation of the educational community.
- Acceptance and valuing of ambiguity in curriculum development.
- Assumption of role-modeling position in relation to enacting curriculum change.
- Development of widening perspective beyond the program level to the professional level.

Faculty/Program Preparation

- Recognition of curriculum as a teacher–student dynamic by creating greater flexibility in timelines and requirements for course decisions, resource allocations, scheduling, and evaluation.
- Acceptance of curriculum work as a critical component of academic life, and of modifications in faculty evaluation criteria and resource allocations.
- Leadership in curriculum inquiry through committee structures and academic environments that value the collective and individual contributions of teacher, student, clinician, and community representatives.
- Advocacy in supporting program autonomy through professional community dialogue, resistance to rigid prescriptions, and valuing of exploration and experimentation.

- Assumption of responsibility to balance needs and interest of accreditation, resources, and curriculum development.

Institution Preparation

- Acceptance of more flexible, less structured definition of program curriculum by decision-making and approval-granting bodies of the university.
- Greater flexibility in resource allocation to support professional programs that are practicum-based.
- Realignment of relative emphasis on teaching, research, and service, to encourage faculty development and research in the area of curriculum development.

Community Preparation

- Creation of flexible, open networks in schools, clinical settings, professional organizations, and academic institutions to encourage regular, consistent interaction related to curriculum development in nursing education.
- Increased profile of "academics," "students," and "clinicians" as an educational community that supports the education of nurses.
- Reexamination of community resources as impacting curriculum development in nursing education.

Professional Organization Preparation

- Agreement to dialogue about greater flexibility in standards and accreditation requirements and procedures.
- Broadening of scope of acceptable criteria for accreditation, allowing greater autonomy and responsibility at the program level.
- Articulated support of exploring innovative ways to ensure public safety and, at the same time, to encourage curriculum flexibility.
- Commitment to assist in establishing a network for nurse educators to support dialogue, publication, and research exchanges related to curriculum issues.

In applying the tenets of the Curriculum Revolution, nurse educators must respond to the multisystem levels that affect and are affected by changes in curriculum inquiry. It is vitally important that careful consideration be given to these areas as an integral part of experimentation. In addition, the examination of application efforts is critical at this stage of development. A strategy to support curriculum research, dialogue around case applications, and interaction among piloting efforts needs to be developed in order to provide an articulated basis for development and improvement in curriculum inquiry. In this way, the education community in nursing can continue to grow and develop within a spirit of creativity, experimentation, flexibility, and interaction.

CONCLUSION

This chapter has attempted to explore the meanings of the Curriculum Revolution by examining its evolution in relation to the caring perspective and mandates. The Curriculum Revolution clearly constitutes a significant turning point in nursing education: it seeks to alter the directions of almost 40 years of Tyler-based curriculum development and to provide the theoretical bases for alternative approaches that are embedded in changes to the traditional dimensions of power, politics, and public policy. At this point, the Curriculum Revolution is being nurtured by a relatively small group of nurse educators. Whether this movement survives and continues to develop, or dies away as an interesting flash in the pan, depends largely on leadership abilities to increase community membership, create structures and processes for interaction and dialogue, support theoretical development, and encourage practice piloting. A commitment to the caring perspective in nursing education offers a powerful potential to revolutionize curriculum development through a restructuring of power, politics, and public policy relationships and, subsequently, to revolutionize the future practice of nursing.

REFERENCES

Allen, D. G. (1990). The Curriculum Revolution: Radical revisioning of nursing education. *Journal of Nursing Education, 29*(7), 312–316.

Appleton, C. (1990). The meaning of human care and the experience of caring in a university school of nursing. In M. Leininger & J. Watson (Eds.), *The caring imperative in education* (pp. 77–94). New York: National League for Nursing Press.

Beck, C. T. (1992). Caring among nursing students. *Nurse Educator, 17*(6), 22–27.

Bevis, E. O. (1973). *Curriculum building in nursing.* St. Louis: Mosby.

Bevis, E. O. (1988). New directions for a new age. In National League for Nursing (Ed.), *Curriculum Revolution: Mandate for change* (pp. 27–52). New York: National League for Nursing Press.

Bevis, E. O. (1989). The curriculum consequences: Aftermath of revolution. In National League for Nursing (Ed.), *Curriculum Revolution: Reconceptualizing nursing education* (pp. 115–134). New York: National League for Nursing Press.

Bevis, E. O. (1990). Has the revolution become the new religion? In National League for Nursing (Ed.), *Curriculum Revolution: Redefining the student–teaching relationship* (pp. 57–66). New York: National League for Nursing Press.

Bevis, E. O., & Clayton, G. (1988). Needed: A new curriculum development design. *Nurse Educator, 13*(4), 14–18.

Bramadat, I. J., & Chalmers, K. I. (1989). Nursing education in Canada: Historical progress—contemporary issues. *Journal of Advanced Nursing, 14*, 719–726.

Chinn, P. L. (1989). Feminist pedagogy in nursing education. In National League for Nursing (Ed.), *Curriculum Revolution: Reconceptualizing nursing education* (pp. 9–24). New York: National League for Nursing Press.

Chinn, P. L. (1990). Gossip: A transformative art for nursing education. *Journal of Nursing Education, 29*(7), 318–321.

Choporian, T. J. (1990). The two worlds of nursing: The one we teach about, the one that is. In National League for Nursing (Ed.), *Curriculum Revolution: Redefining the student–teaching relationship* (pp. 21–36). New York: National League for Nursing Press.

Conley, V. C. (1973). *Curriculum and instruction in nursing.* Boston: Little, Brown.

deTornyay, R. (1990). The Curriculum Revolution. *Journal of Nursing Education, 29*(7), 292–294.

Diekelmann, N. (1989). The nursing curriculum: Lived experiences of students. In National League for Nursing (Ed.), *Curriculum Revolution: Reconceptualizing nursing education* (pp. 25–42). New York: National League for Nursing Press.

Diekelmann, N. (1990). Nursing education: Caring, dialogue, and practice. *Journal of Nursing Education, 29*(7), 300–305.

Diekelmann, N. (1992). Learning-as-testing: A Heideggerian hermeneutical analysis of the lived experiences of students and teachers in nursing. *Advances in Nursing Science, 14*(3), 72–83.

Diekelmann, N. (1993). Behavioral pedagogy: A Heideggerian hermeneutical analysis of the lived experiences of students and teachers in baccalaureate education. *Journal of Nursing Education, 32*(6), 245–254.

Donley, Sr. R. (1989). Curriculum Revolution: Heeding the voice of change. In National League for Nursing (Ed.), *Curriculum Revolution: Reconceptualizing nursing education* (pp. 1–8). New York: National League for Nursing Press.

Halldorsdottir, S. (1990). The essential structure of a caring and an uncaring encounter with a teacher: The perspective of the nursing student. In M. Leininger & J. Watson (Eds.), *The caring imperative in education* (pp. 95–108). New York: National League for Nursing Press.

Hughes, L. (1992). Faculty–student interactions and the student-perceived climate for caring. *Advances in Nursing Science, 14*(3), 60–71.

Hughes, L. (1993). Peer group interactions and the student-perceived climate for caring. *Journal of Nursing Education, 32*(2), 78–83.

King, E. M. (1974). Curriculum design for the 1980's. In National League for Nursing (Ed.), *Curriculum relevance within a changing health care system* (pp. 43–66). New York: National League for Nursing Press.

King, M. K. (1970). The development of university nursing education. In M. Q. Innis (Ed.), *Nursing education in a changing society* (pp. 67–85). Toronto: University of Toronto Press.

Miller, B. K., Haber, J., & Byrne, M. W. (1990). The experience of caring in the teaching–learning process of nursing education: Student and teacher perspectives. In M. Leininger & J. Watson (Eds.), *The caring imperative in education* (pp. 125–135). New York: National League for Nursing Press.

Moccia, P. (1990). No sire: It's a revolution. *Journal of Nursing Education, 29*(7), 307–311.

Murdock, J. (1983). Curriculum development in nursing: Historical perspective. In M. B. White (Ed.), *Curriculum development from a nursing model: The crisis theory framework* (pp. 1–25). New York: Springer.

Murdock, J. E. (1986). Evolution of the nursing curriculum. *Journal of Nursing History, 2*(1), 16–35.

Mussallem, H. K. (1965). *Nursing education in Canada.* Ottawa: Royal Commission on Health Services.

National League for Nursing. (1988, October). Curriculum Revolution: Mandate for change. *Nursing and Health Care,* p. 421.

Roach, Sr. M. S. (1991). Creating communities of caring. In National League for Nursing (Ed.), *Curriculum Revolution: Community building and activism* (pp. 123–138). New York: National League for Nursing Press.

Tanner, C. (1988, October). Curriculum Revolution: The practice mandate. *Nursing and Health Care,* pp. 427–430.

Tanner, C. A. (1990a). Introduction. In National League for Nursing (Ed.), *Curriculum Revolution: Redefining the student–teaching relationship* (pp. 1–4). New York: National League for Nursing Press.

Tanner, C. A. (1990b). Reflections on the Curriculum Revolution. *Journal of Nursing Education*, 29(7), 295–299.

Tyler, R. W. (1949). *Basic principles of curriculum and instruction*. Chicago: University of Chicago Press.

Valiga, T. M. (1988). Curriculum outcomes and cognitive development: New perspectives for nursing education. In National League for Nursing (Ed.), *Curriculum Revolution: Mandate for change* (pp. 177–200). New York: National League for Nursing Press.

Watson, J. (1988, October). Human caring as moral context for nursing education. *Nursing and Health Care*, pp. 423–425.

Watson, J. (1990). Transformation in nursing: Bringing care back to health care. In National League for Nursing (Ed.), *Curriculum Revolution: Redefining the student–teaching relationship* (pp. 15–20). New York: National League for Nursing Press.

13

Professional Nurse Caring: Surviving the Transition to the Workplace

Lesley M. Wilkes
Marianne C. Wallis

. . . caring is not unique to any particular profession. . . . Caring rather may be considered unique in nursing. (Roach, 1992, p. 47)

As nurses and educators, we reflect on the imperative of developing caring attributes in students of nursing and the changes in these attributes that may occur once students enter the workforce. Our original work on this topic indicated that students of nursing have developed attributes of caring by the end of their university studies (Wilkes & Wallis, 1993). Further study revealed that these caring attributes developed throughout the course of study (Wallis & Wilkes, 1993). In doing this work, however, we have been continuously confronted by the often-voiced concern, from individuals in practice settings, that new graduates do not display these unique caring attributes. The purpose of this chapter is to describe how attributes of caring change as the nurse's environment changes from the university to the workplace.

LITERATURE REVIEW

Professional Nurse Caring

The human science literature focusing on care and caring is copious and diverse. Readers keen to explore different perspectives on caring could look at literature from many different disciplines. Caring as a concept or construct has been explored philosophically (Heidegger, 1962; Mayeroff, 1972), psychologically (Rogers & Stevens, 1967), sociologically (Gilligan, 1982; Noddings, 1984), anthropologically (Leininger, 1981), historically (Gustafson, 1984), and from many different nursing perspectives (see Morse, Bottorff, Neander, & Solberg, 1991). Also, in recent years, the study of moral reasoning and ethics has, largely under the influence of feminist social psychology theory, expanded to consider the place of caring in ethics.

The debate surrounding caring has, more recently, concentrated on eliciting caring as a distinctive aspect of professional nursing (Leininger, 1984; Watson, 1979). Leininger (1988, p. 9) differentiates among "generic caring," "professional caring," and "professional nurse caring." Generic caring is her name for the caring that characterizes many human relationships—a mother for her child, one friend for another, or neighbors to each other. Professional caring, which goes beyond generic caring, is seen in a number of the helping professions. Professional nurse caring is the caring that is unique to nursing and requires cognitive, affective, and motor skills. Professional nurse caring is said to be directed toward sustaining and improving the health and well-being of clients (Leininger, 1988). It is said to be, variously, "a humanistic–scientific combination" (Watson, 1979); "culturally diverse and universal" (Leininger, 1988); "a special way of being, knowing and doing with the goal of protection and enhancement of human dignity" (Watson, 1988); and "the synthesis of a motor component, cognitive component and affective component and a cultural component" (Metcalfe, 1990).

A Model of Professional Nurse Caring from the Perspective of Student Nurses

In previous work, we developed a theory of professional nurse caring from the perspective of university nursing students (Wallis & Wilkes, 1993; Wilkes & Wallis, 1993). From the perspective of students, there seems to be a momentary pinnacle of professional nurse caring that they all strive for but do not all necessarily achieve.

The model attempts to bind the core of caring—compassion—with a number of "caring actions" specific to the nurse. Compassion, as the core of caring, is seen as: to love, to have and share feelings, to be a friend, and to be concerned for others. This core of caring is seen in a number of attributes that are actualized in the students' nursing of patients (clients) through:

- Communicating (listening, talking, explaining, touching, educating, expressing feelings);
- Providing comfort (doing, assisting, helping);
- Being competent (assessing, watching for cues, having knowledge and skills, being responsible and professional);
- Being committed (doing, loving, showing no bias, "being there");
- Having conscience (attending, giving the person dignity and respect, treating as oneself);
- Being confident (knowing what to do, without hesitation);
- Being courageous (advocating for a person's needs and rights to treatment, intervening for and with the person).

The first of these caring actions is not only an actualization of professional nurse caring but often forms the link between the core of caring (compassion) and the other caring actions. In this way, communicating constitutes an important medium for the expression of the caring actions.

This model of professional nurse caring can be seen as a momentary pinnacle of the whole experience of caring to which students could aspire, but there were overt and obvious changes in their perceptions over the three years of their university education. A beginning student of nursing brings some caring attributes, such as compassion, to his or her entry into nursing. Over the course of undergraduate study, all students develop and add to their personal attributes, but in differing degrees (Wallis & Wilkes, 1993; Wilkes & Wallis, 1993).

This professionalization of human caring involves the development of a capacity to care in light of specific roles and responsibilities (Roach, 1984). As a person moves from being a student to being a registered nurse, the literature postulates that his or her roles and responsibilities change.

Transition to Graduate Nurse

Benner (1984) states that new graduate nurses enter the workplace as novices. They have been taught objective facts in preparation for the experience, and they have learned rules to guide their practice. However, the graduates have no experience with many practice situations. They have provided care to a small number of patients but have not assumed the full duties and responsibilities of a registered nurse. Owens's (1991) study of the perceptions of caring among undergraduate students in a three-year diploma-in-nursing program in Wollongong, New South Wales, Australia, revealed that the students found caring a difficult concept to describe. They stated that they did not talk about caring in the classroom; instead, they felt constructs of caring came from the clinical setting. It is important to note that, for university students in Australia, clinical practice is undertaken in a very safe environment with an educator present. Accountability for timelines and priorities is the responsibility of registered nurses employed in the setting, not the students.

Kramer (1974) suggested that new graduates, in the initial few months of practice and in response to the shock of their new environment, often disregard values developed during their tertiary education. Australian studies of graduate nurses from college/university programs (Bates, 1993; Goldsworthy, Pickhaver, & Young, 1984) have shown that the graduates manifested some aspects of this reality shock.

Jenifer Harvey (1988), a graduate from a three-year diploma-in-nursing program in New South Wales, Australia, relates that the nurse graduate enters a world of challenges and turmoil. Her experience has revealed the issues that confront the graduate: the mixed attitudes of registered nurses trained in hospital programs; the questioning by the general public as to whether the tertiary education for nurses contains too little clinical training; and the new experience of shift work. Another Australian graduate, who completed study at a later date, states, "[our education at University] is only a starting point . . . [it] . . . has provided us with a good theoretical background and it's up to us to put it into practice, but you need time to do so. After working for several months things fall into place (even all those theories)" (Murdoch, 1993, p. 24).

Graduate nurses move from the safe environment experienced by the student to that of the worker–registered nurse. They are now employees and have become accountable for their performance. Their responsibilities and roles have changed. The question arose: How do professional nurse caring attributes change as the environment changes?

CASE STUDIES OF FOUR FIRST-YEAR NURSING GRADUATES

The model described earlier in this chapter was developed with students in a university environment. As an adjunct to this study, we wanted to address whether these caring attributes changed as the student moved into the work environment as a graduate registered nurse. Four case studies of nurses one year postgraduation were used to examine the changes that occurred in the caring attributes displayed by these nurses. Because each graduate's experience is different, there is no aim to generalize from these data. The four graduates had originally participated in the research project that led to the development of the model.

Data Collection

Qualitative data were collected using a lived experience focus. The four participants, all women, completed a written survey in November 1990, at the end of their three-year Diploma in Health Science (Nursing) program, which qualified them for registration as nurses in New South Wales, Australia. The survey consisted of two questions:

1.   What is the meaning of caring to you?

2.   Describe an incident during your last practicum [clinical] in which you perceive you were caring to a patient/client.

The participants were interviewed after completing this questionnaire. A second interview took place in April 1991, three months after they commenced employment, and a final interview was conducted in April 1992. The interviews, which used a semistructured format, were audiotaped with the participants' permission. In the first interview, the interviewer requested elaboration of contextual themes that emerged from the participants' survey, and prompted them when necessary. In the second and subsequent interviews, each participant was asked to describe recent caring incidents and to discuss how she viewed these incidents. The participant was also asked about noncaring. In the final interview, she was asked whether she thought her caring had changed over the past year.

Data Analysis

All texts of surveys and transcribed interviews of the four graduates were examined and coded by the researchers for emerging themes, with the assistance of the Ethnograph computer program (Seidel, Kjolseth, & Seymour, 1988). These themes were then compared with the prior model, and similarities and differences were explored.

The Four Case Studies

Nurse A.   Nurse A had only community and nursing-home experience over the 12 months. She had a general notion of caring as "being nice and touching, doing things for people," which was reflected in all three interviews. In her last interview, she stated that to be caring was to make the "patient happy." This was the only construct of caring that she emphasized at this time. Nurse A stated that the reason for this emphasis might be that she herself was much happier as she had just remarried.

Her concern for patients was strongly expressed at her first interview, when she stated that caring was:

> . . . being generally concerned for others because caring goes beyond doing what's ordered, doesn't it!

In this first interview, she also spoke of giving time to a particular patient:

> . . . wanting to and making time to be with a lady having chemotherapy . . . who seemed to me to want company to ease the anxiety and the boredom I sat and talked to her . . . she just wanted to have a chat.

At the time of her second interview, Nurse A was doing mainly physical care for patients in the home. As a result, her articulation of care was mostly described in these terms. She did note one incident where she took extra effort to do something for a particular patient. However, Nurse A still expressed her caring through a sense of "niceness":

> I just try to pamper her . . . I try to do nice things for her. She loves me to kiss her goodbye and kisses me hello.

This last quote also indicates a relationship in which the nurse was expecting and getting some rewards.

Nurse B.   Nurse B was working as a registered nurse in a large private hospital. Throughout the 12 months of the study, she was employed in a medical/surgical cardiac ward. Nurse B's caring attributes varied markedly over the year that separated the interviews. In the first interview, Nurse B clearly expressed that caring entailed compassion mediated through communication:

> . . . even little things like putting their flowers in a vase or going in and talking to them . . . even when you're really busy you can still talk to them while you're doing things . . . and that's all part of caring as far as I am concerned.

An incident that occurred just before she graduated, and secondhand experience related by her preceptor, had caused Nurse B to question the nature of commitment as a caring attribute:

> I became attached to both of them, they really were a nice couple. When her husband died I was really "down" about it for a while and I thought . . . well, I don't want to get into that stuff . . . get that attached any more.

When reminded of this patient at the second interview, Nurse B reiterated that she had been very attached, the death of the patient's husband had upset her, and she would avoid attachment like that in the future. However, she was able to give examples of commitment within a caring relationship that showed not only a more professional relationship emerging but also the genesis of other caring attributes, such as competence and responsibility:

> Caring is a whole lot different than as a student, because it's on a broader spectrum . . . .

> . . . you've got the authority to do things . . . .

In the first interview, Nurse B linked the idea of caring with the nurse's being rewarded or feeling good. By the time of the last interview, the issues of commitment and conscience within caring had assumed great importance. The caring experience that Nurse B spent most time describing was related to a difficult and unpopular patient. This time, Nurse B chose to describe how another nurse had shown commitment, compassion, competence, concern, and conscience through communication:

> . . . Nurse X will sit and talk to her for ages . . . she'll leave her other work or she'll stay back . . . . She puts in the effort. . . . The lady just screams and

*cries all the time but Nurse X will always go in and say hello. . . . Nurse X
has been nursing for a while and she's got her time management down pat and
everything but it's more . . . she can really soothe this lady. Nurse X sticks at
it for so long whereas I think, "Oh, let her go."*

By the end of the third interview, Nurse B was reflecting on her perception
of change in her own professional nurse caring. She was clear that her caring
had changed enormously from the time she worked as an assistant in nursing
while still at the University:

*I know I'm a lot more caring than I was then. It was so unprofessional, you
just had to get it all done . . . I suppose getting older, having experience, the
patients have changed me. Probably I've got better . . . I don't say better at
caring, but even if they're cranky they still need to be cared for. They probably show it in a different way.*

One other aspect of caring that Nurse B was keen to comment on in the third
interview was how to teach caring. Nurse B was adamant:

The only thing that made a huge impact on me at [University] was my educators.

When questioned further, Nurse B felt that her educators had taught her to
care not only by modeling in the clinical setting but, almost more importantly,
by being present as concerned, caring persons in the educational setting:

*I found the nursing lecturers were a lot more caring about us than the non-
nursing lecturers. . . . Like even just the fact that they cared about you . . .
you thought, "They'd be a good nurse."*

Nurse B concluded her last interview with reference to what was the best
thing about caring in nursing. For her, receiving thanks for her caring, being
remembered by the patient even if she had not been very demonstrative, was:

*. . . [what] brings you back down to earth . . . that's what's nice about
nursing.*

Nurse C.   Nurse C obtained a position as a registered nurse in a large private hospital with a strong Christian denominational ethos. She entered the "new graduate" program at the hospital and rotated through three wards, spending four months working on each.

In contrast to Nurse B, Nurse C's caring attributes did not change, although their scope increased markedly. Nurse C's widening experience served to give her more opportunities to demonstrate professional nurse caring. However, the basic parameters were in place much earlier. Nurse C's overriding caring attribute came across as compassion. How this compassion was mediated through communication was clear from the first interview:

> Yes, I try to make sure that I am there for them if they need to talk or need to ask something. Like when you just go in to do their care, often you just touch their hand or smile . . . it lets them know they can always ask.

By the third interview, the compassion and communication were matched by a competence born of experience, which meant that the communication could also be used to teach. Nurse C described her care of a patient who had been newly diagnosed with cancer:

> I nursed her most of the time . . . so that was like sitting down and talking to her . . . even if I wasn't looking after her that day. She needed to discuss her options and things like that.

As Nurse C progressed through the experiences of her first year as an RN, attributes of compassion, communication, commitment, concern, taking time, and being rewarded expanded to include increasing confidence and competence. During the second interview, Nurse C described how she had been sent to an unfamiliar ward to relieve:

> . . . but it was good in a way because it gave me a look at total patient nursing, so it gave me a bit more confidence in that I can do medications and that I can totally care for a patient without someone else taking the responsibility.

In her third interview, Nurse C described two incidents; in the latter, her increasing competence became apparent even while her confidence was low.

She was describing how a patient suddenly became critically ill, and, although she questioned whether she could have done more, eventually she said:

> We had done everything we could . . . we had called the resident, called the doctors. There was nothing more we could have done. . . . Sometimes you can miss the patient's needs trying to give them the medical backup that they need. But I think we were quite good because there was a couple of us, so there was always someone with the patient.

Following this incident, Nurse C expressed the view that supporting and being supported by other nurses was an important aspect of caring:

> . . . giving the other staff involved feedback and support. . . . Then the NUM [Nurse Unit Manager] followed it up through the week and just asked if we were alright . . . and things like that . . . so it was good.

One incident illustrates Nurse C's courage. In an unusual circumstance where she was not feeling confident, she managed to overcome her fear to care for the patient:

> Well, I did find it very frightening because I had only been on the ward for two months . . . I think you give more to the patient at that time, than to yourself. You sort of use all your resources that aren't tied up in your adrenalin running and trying to get everything done. I think you give more to the patient, so it's more emotionally draining on you as well because your extra bit of energy is going towards holding their hand or letting them know what is going on.

Interestingly, Nurse C also believed that as her professional nurse caring developed so did her capacity for generic caring.

> You think, well, if I can do this for this person (patient), I should be able to do it for my family as well.

Nurse C felt that caring could best be taught through role modeling and that her capacity to care is reduced when she is stressed. When Nurse C would visit her family again:

That's when you need to build up your resources again or you won't be very caring . . . Mum and Dad are always there . . . and my other family . . . and spending time with them just picks me up.

Nurse D.   Prior to studying for a Diploma in Health Science (Nursing), Nurse D had worked as an assistant in nursing for 13 years, mainly in the area of palliative care. During her first year as a registered nurse she completed the requirements for a Bachelor Degree in Nursing.

Initially, Nurse D worked on a general ward, in a public hospital (250-bed capacity) southwest of Sydney. Twelve months later, she assumed the position of her choice in a coronary care/intensive care unit at the same hospital. Nurse D's perceptions of caring were set at the first interview, when she expressed compassion in the sense of sharing with the patient and being available:

. . . sharing that feeling with the patient, or feeling sorry for that person during whatever time that person is with you.

This concept of time was very important in Nurse D's sense of caring and was reiterated in the second and third interviews. Talking about an older woman in the surgical ward where Nurse D was working at six months, she said:

I made time to go and say hello . . . because of the time constraint of nursing I didn't have time to give her special care, but when I had done my work I'd go to her and spend some time with her.

Also, at the third interview:

[caring] . . . is being there, being nonjudgmental. First of all, it's spending an extra couple of minutes. It makes a big difference.

At the third interview, Nurse D reflected on the fact that even though her idea of caring was no different, she was more confident in her practice because she had the background knowledge, through her nursing courses, to be more effective in her care:

Before, when I worked [that is, as an assistant in nursing], I didn't understand a lot of the anatomy and physiology and how people are affected mentally by illness. I have a greater understanding now, and this makes me more aware.

At her last interview, Nurse D was more aware of the need for nurses to understand the cultural differences in caring as perceived by patients. She recalled a specific case of a man with a massive heart attack who was very frightened and needed a lot of extra attention:

> He needed constant reinforcement, and people need to know about culture . . . he was Lebanese . . . and the family is very important. They want to be there all the time. This sometimes becomes a problem if you don't recognize it.

REFLECTION ON THE CASE STUDIES

Nursing students develop attributes of professional nurse caring in an environment that is structured and supportive. This development is fostered when students are not responsible for or accountable for the professional nurse caring they provide. From these case studies, it becomes clear that each person brought to her first year as a registered nurse different past experience. During the first year as a graduate nurse, further unique experiences of life and of working as a registered nurse influenced each person's expression of professional nurse caring. When the graduates from this study entered the workplace, their responsibilities changed and, initially, this appeared to alter their ability to put into practice attributes of professional nurse caring.

One predominant concern of the graduates was the availability of time to communicate with patients when so many other things were happening and/or the patient was in crisis. This exemplifies the importance of communicating as a caring action and as an expression of caring for the nurse; that is, caring as compassion shines through communication.

This need to prioritize activities and make decisions that incorporate the "good" of more than one patient at a time was a feature of the reality shock of new graduates described by Kramer (1974) and, in an Australian study, by Bates (1993). Both authors told how new graduates often found it traumatic and disillusioning to face the ethical dilemmas arising out of having to defer one patient's need to communicate, in favor of meeting responsibilities to a number of other patients. Many of the graduates cited in these studies had difficulty in reconciling their experience of the practical environment with the theoretical tenets of their place of education. In the university, they were encouraged to take time and be with the patient. The supportive environment around them meant that, by the end of their course, they were able to do this (Wilkes & Wallis, 1993). Once they had graduated, their support was less, their responsibilities greater, and the time they had available to spend with individual patients was limited.

As the year progressed, the graduates in this study began to own the hospital as their environment. They became confident and competent, and again began to have time to spend with the patient. Caring attributes described in the earlier model (Figure 13–1) again surfaced. This pattern may be related to Gadamer's (1976/1981) philosophy of practice, in which he contends that practical wisdom is different with *techne* (the acquired skill of the expert). Practical wisdom gives the practitioner the ability to prioritize activity in relation to the "good" of the action. Thus, as Bishop and Scudder (1990) contend:

> . . . *nurses who possess practical wisdom would examine priorities in nursing and make decisions about the use of time on the basis of that which is choiceworthy . . . and this decision making would not originate from outside practice but choices would be made on the basis of the good at which practice aims.* (p. 74)

These authors go on to suggest that this practical wisdom is informed by a nursing ethic (Bishop & Scudder, 1990). The researchers in the present study contend that this nursing ethic is the ethic of professional nurse caring, and that the graduates in this study had not yet fully developed this practical wisdom to direct their professional nurse caring.

Bishop & Scudder (1990) maintain that practical wisdom and the ethic that informs it can only be taught in the clinical setting. The graduates all believed that they had learned about caring and the ethics that underpin it in the clinical setting. However, they all cited their spiritual beliefs, personal development, or family as the rich soil in which the seed of caring was originally planted. It is also interesting to note that Nurse B believed that she learned about caring from the nursing lecturers both in the University environment and in the clinical setting. This supports the results of a study, conducted in North America, which found that nursing students who had experienced caring from faculty members "wished to reach out to someone else through caring" (Beck, 1991, p. 21).

REFERENCES

Bates, W. (1993). The difficulties of applied practice experienced by recently graduated tertiary nursing students in their first six months of employment in a major public hospital. *Proceedings of the National Conference on Research in Nursing: Turning Points.* South Australia: Centre For Nursing Research.

Beck, C. T. (1991). How students perceive faculty caring: A phenomenological study. *Nurse Educator, 16*(5), 18–22.

Benner, P. D. (1984). *From novice to expert: Excellence and power in clinical nursing practice.* Menlo Park, CA: Addison-Wesley.

Bishop, A. H., & Scudder, J. R. (1990). *The practical, moral, and personal sense of nursing: A phenomenological philosophy of practice.* Albany, NY: SUNY Press.

Gadamer, H. G. (1981). *Reason in the age of science* (F. G. Lawrence, Trans.). Cambridge, MA: MIT Press. (Original work published 1976)

Gilligan, C. (1982). *In a different voice: Psychological theory and women's development.* Cambridge, MA: Harvard University Press.

Goldsworthy, L., Pickhaver, A., & Young, W. (1984). *They're different somehow.* Adelaide, South Australia: South Australian College of Advanced Education.

Gustafson, W. (1984). Motivational and historical aspects of care and nursing. In M. M. Leininger (Ed.), *Care: The essence of nursing and health.* Thorofare, NJ: Slack.

Harvey, J. (1988). Life's not easy when you're first through a course, but . . . . *Australian Journal of Advanced Nursing, 5*(4), 19–21.

Heidegger, M. (1962). *Being and time* (J. Macquarie & E. Robinson, Trans.). New York: Harper & Row. (Original work published 1927)

Kramer, M. (1974). *Reality shock: Transitions of students of nursing.* Menlo Park, CA: Addison-Wesley.

Leininger, M. (1981). *Caring: An essential human need.* Thorofare, NJ: Slack.

Leininger, 1984? (p. 289)

Leininger, M. M. (1988). *Caring: An essential human need.* Detroit: Wayne State University Press.

Mayeroff, M. (1972). *On caring.* New York: Harper & Row.

Metcalfe, S. (1990). Knowing care in the clinical field context: An educator's point of view. In M. Leininger & J. Watson (Eds.), *The caring imperative in education.* New York: National League for Nursing Press.

Morse, J. M., Bottorff, J., Neander, W., & Solberg, S. (1991). Comparative analysis of conceptualisations and theories of caring. *Image: The Journal of Nursing Scholarship, 23*(2), 119–126.

Murdoch, F. (1993). Surviving the transition: From university student to registered nurse. *Australian Nursing Journal, 1*(5), 21, 24.

Noddings, N. (1984). *Caring: A feminine approach to ethics and moral education.* Berkeley: University of California Press.

Owens, J. (1990). *Nursing students' constructs of caring.* Unpublished master's thesis, University of Wollongong.

Roach, M. S. (1984). *Caring: The human mode of being—Implications for nursing.* Toronto: University of Toronto.

Roach, M. S. (1992). *The human act of caring: A blueprint for the health professions* (rev. ed.). Ottawa: Canadian Hospitals Association.

Rogers, C. R., & Stevens, B. (1967). *Person to person: The problem of being human.* New York: Pocket Books.

Seidel, J. V., Kjolseth, R., & Seymour, E. (1988). *The ethnograph: A user's guide.* Corvallis, OR: Qualis.

Wallis, M. C., & Wilkes, L. M. (1993). *A journey to professional nurse caring.* Paper presented at NSW Nurses Research Interest Group Annual Conference, Sydney.

Watson, J. (1979). *Nursing: The philosophy and science of caring.* Boston: Little, Brown.

Watson, J. (1988). New dimensions of human caring theory. *Nursing Science Quarterly, 1*(4), 175–181.

Wilkes, L. M., & Wallis, M. C. (1993). The five C's of Caring: the lived experiences of student nurses. *Australian Journal of Advanced Nursing, 11*(1), 19–25.